Understanding and Managing Your Child's Food Allergies

A Johns Hopkins Press Health Book

Understanding and Managing

YOUR CHILD'S FOOD ALLERGIES

SCOTT H. SICHERER, M.D.

THE JOHNS HOPKINS UNIVERSITY PRESS BALTIMORE

Notes to the Reader

This book is not meant to substitute for medical care of people with allergies, and treatment should not be based solely on its contents. Instead, treatment must be developed in a dialogue between the individual and his or her physician. This book has been written to help with that dialogue. The author and publisher are not responsible for any adverse consequences resulting from the use of information in this book.

The individual case histories in this book are derived from composites of many patient encounters. None of the case histories represents a particular person or patient. Names, ages, and identifying information have been changed to protect privacy.

Drug dosage: The author and publisher have made reasonable efforts to determine that the selection and dosage of drugs discussed in this text conform to the practices of the general medical community. The medications described do not necessarily have specific approval by the U.S. Food and Drug Administration for use in the diseases and dosages for which they are recommended. In view of ongoing research, changes in governmental regulations, and the constant flow of information relating to drug therapy and drug reactions, the reader is urged to check the package insert of each drug for any change in indications and dosage and for warnings and precautions. This is particularly important when the recommended agent is a new and/or infrequently used drug.

Printed in the United States of America on acid-free paper
9 8 7 6 5 4 3 2 1

The Johns Hopkins University Press
2715 North Charles Street
Baltimore, Maryland 21218-4363
www.press.jhu.edu

The Food Allergy Action Plan on pages 288–89 is reprinted with permission from the Food Allergy & Anaphylaxis Network (www.foodallergy.org).

Library of Congress Cataloging-in-Publication Data

Sicherer, Scott H.
Understanding and managing your child's food allergies / Scott H. Sicherer.
p. cm.
Includes bibliographical references (p.) and index.
ISBN 0-8018-8491-8 (hardcover : alk. paper) — ISBN 0-8018-8492-6 (pbk. : alk. paper)
1. Food allergy in children. I. Title.
RJ386.5.S53 2006
618.92′975—dc22 2006005261

A catalog record for this book is available from the British Library.

Contents

To the Reader

This book is dedicated first to families whose children are living with food allergies. I've had thousands of interactions with children who have food allergies and their siblings, parents, and grandparents. You taught me, through your successes, what to teach others. You taught me, through your difficulties, what pitfalls to teach others to watch out for and how to overcome them. You taught me, through your quest to better manage life with food allergies, what research to undertake, and what you and others need to know to better manage life with food allergies. You taught me that in knowledge there is both power and comfort and that by understanding your child's food allergy, you, your child, and those who care for your child can better manage this illness. Through words and actions, you asked me to write this book. It is my pleasure and privilege to have done that—to give you a place to find accurate, timely, and detailed information on every aspect of your child's food allergies. I sincerely hope this book provides you with the information and tools you need to understand and manage your child's food allergies.

Of course, the information in this book would not exist without the work and influence of many people. So, I also dedicate this book to Hugh A. Sampson, M.D., who is not only a colleague, friend, and mentor but also an individual who can be credited with bringing food allergy into focus as a medical disorder in need of research toward finding a cure. To Anne Muñoz-Furlong, founder of the Food Allergy & Anaphylaxis Network, who has, along with her husband, Terry, a wonderful team of dedicated staff, and a remarkable board of medical advisors, made triumphant advances in increasing awareness and improving life for those with food allergies. To Sally Noone, R.N., and Shideh Mofidi, R.D., at the Jaffe Food Allergy Institute at

Mount Sinai for their constant support. To Robert A. Wood, M.D., for his mentoring, for his careful review of this book, and for his kind suggestions. To my many medical colleagues at Mount Sinai, and to researchers worldwide, who have already made numerous remarkable discoveries and are poised to find treatments and cures for food allergies. To the Food Allergy Initiative, for proving that a group of concerned parents can promote research and awareness, and with resounding success. To the Jaffe family, for their foresight in establishing a Food Allergy Institute. And, finally, to my wife, Mati, and children, Andrew, Zachary, Maya, Sydnee, and Cassaddee . . . for everything.

Foreword

Dr. Sicherer is a rare combination of brains, compassion, understanding, and practicality. Parents will want to have him as their child's allergist. I am lucky to count him as a friend and mentor.

As one of the world's experts on food allergy, Dr. Sicherer is always willing to listen and gain new insight from his patients and their parents. Anyone who has attended one of his lectures knows they are lively, funny, and filled with information. *Understanding and Managing Your Child's Food Allergies* is a combination of all those things. This book encompasses answers to the thousands of questions he's been asked by parents around the country. He has given generously of his vast understanding of this issue and of his time to help families living with food allergies.

His explanations of various food allergy–associated diseases and diagnostic tests are complete and easy to understand. The section on emotional concerns acknowledges what so many individuals living with food allergies know: it affects the entire family and can sometimes be extremely stressful. This section provides helpful strategies for reducing the emotional toll. In the final section, Dr. Sicherer offers a snapshot of what scientists around the world are doing to help tackle food allergy, giving us all hope for a brighter future.

A diagnosis of food allergy can be overwhelming. It is not uncommon for parents to arrive home from the doctor's office with many questions they wished they had asked. Dr. Sicherer's book is a reference tool that belongs in everyone's bookcase. In the beginning, you will undoubtedly turn to it for answers to your questions about allergy testing, outgrowing food allergy, and managing allergies at childcare or in school. In the years to come, it will offer confirmation that you are doing the right thing as your child develops from infancy to the teen years and beyond.

Anne Muñoz-Furlong
Founder and CEO
The Food Allergy & Anaphylaxis Network

Introduction

Over the past twenty-five years, I have had the privilege of witnessing and participating in a remarkable evolution in our understanding of food allergy. When I began my research in food allergy in the early 1980s, I approached the disorder by applying my background in detailed scientific methods. Initially I was encouraged to explore this area by Dr. Susan Dees at Duke University. Later, I became fascinated with the field because of experiences with my second daughter, who had food allergies, eczema, and later asthma, and by the increasing number of families and children I cared for in my clinical practice. In those early years, I was reluctant to admit to my research colleagues that I was focusing my research on food allergy. The reason for my trepidation was that food allergy in those days was considered not a "real disease" but rather a problem of little consequence. Part of the reason for this misunderstanding about food allergy was that many people attributed a variety of problems to foods that were never scientifically proved to be related. At the same time, people were not recognizing allergic diseases that actually were caused or worsened by foods. Although everyone acknowledged that a food could cause a severe allergic reaction, the life-threatening nature of this allergy was not well appreciated.

In the mid-1970s, the field of food allergy emerged from scientific uncertainty in part because of the work of Drs. Charles May and Allan Bock, who emphasized the need to use a diagnostic procedure called a double-blind, placebo-controlled oral food challenge (just one of the procedures discussed in this book). This test brought objectivity to the diagnosis of food allergy by eliminating patients' and physicians' preconceived notions. In my research work, this procedure fostered incredible scientific advances to improve the diagnosis and treatment of food allergy. Food allergy became "real," was now viewed as a medical illness worthy of attention, and was acknowledged as a field of allergy in need of more research.

Although the emergence of food allergy from the "dark ages" and into a time of scientific exploration was exciting, the past two decades have unfortunately witnessed an alarming increase in food allergy and other allergic diseases. For reasons we do not fully understand, allergic diseases have become more common, particularly in westernized societies. Our studies estimate that 11 million Americans now have food allergy, and about 5 million who suffer are children. Children are experiencing more food allergies that persist longer than when I began to study this disease. The burden of living with food allergy remains largely untold and underappreciated. Care requires constant dietary caution and the readiness to treat severe allergic reactions. Despite increasing awareness, this disease is sometimes fatal.

The increase in food-allergic disease has been disheartening, but the challenges to improve life for those affected are being met. Over a decade ago, Anne Muñoz-Furlong established the Food Allergy & Anaphylaxis Network (FAAN), which has become a tremendous resource for every aspect of living with food allergy. FAAN's numerous triumphs have resonated through government agencies, legislation, industry, and various health care organizations. FAAN has become a model for similar groups globally. The Food Allergy Initiative in New York and the Jaffe Food Allergy Research Institute established the precedent that parents and the public can affect research on food allergy by raising funds and stimulating national funding agencies to follow suit, increasing research spending in this important area. Remarkable advances have been made, understanding has increased, and the future is looking brighter. But there has been a missing piece.

The simultaneous increase in the number of people with food allergies and in the amount of information now available on food allergy has outpaced our ability to teach parents, children, and caregivers what we have learned. Parents and other caregivers are often confused and cannot find reliable information with sufficient details about a child's food allergies. These individuals have burning questions and concerns. For many of these concerns, we now have clear answers. Where the right answer is unclear, we have plenty of information to help while research is under way. This book is an amazing compilation of the essential information needed to work with your doctor, discuss your child's food allergy with other caregivers and your child, and, ultimately, provide your child with the best care possible. It is the only resource I know of that provides timely, accurate, and accessible information on every medical aspect of food allergy.

In this book, Dr. Sicherer has culled his extensive experience and provided the reader vast information in a format that is readable and easily understandable. He has provided both basic medical information and tips on such everyday issues as visiting the allergist, dealing with schools and restaurants, and navigating the supermarket. As an internationally recognized leader in food allergy education and research, Dr. Sicherer has been at the cutting edge of clinical and social issues of food allergy. As a lecturer, he has had countless experiences discussing food allergy not only with children but also with parents, school nurses, camp directors, food-service employees, pediatricians, allergists, and many others involved in the care of children with food allergies. He has distilled these experiences to address issues you may have encountered or wondered about, as well as those you may not yet have considered.

Though this book is focused toward parents, the information is so comprehensive and timely that it is truly "required reading" for physicians, teachers, school nurses, camp personnel, and everyone who plays a role in caring for children with food allergies. It will help them to understand and more effectively manage a child's food allergies. I will certainly keep a copy of this book in my clinic and recommend it to everyone who is dealing with food allergies.

Hugh A. Sampson, M.D.
Director
The Jaffe Food Allergy Institute

Understanding and Managing Your Child's Food Allergies

PART I

THE MANY FACES OF FOOD ALLERGY

Sally is a happy and playful 5-year-old. She seems perfectly healthy and giggles as I joke with her during her visit to my office. Last week, Sally accidentally ate her friend's chocolate chip cookie instead of her own oatmeal raisin cookie. Sally has a cow's milk allergy. The few innocent bites of that cookie resulted in a severe allergic reaction, a frightening experience of an itchy rash, a face swollen beyond recognition, and breathing trouble. Thankfully, a quick shot of medicine and a trip to the emergency room eased her discomfort—and may have saved her life.

Even after a decade of caring for children with food allergies and conducting research studies in the field of food allergy, I find it hard to fathom that a small bite of food can cause sudden, severe reactions that threaten a child's life. It's almost unimaginable that food, which we depend on for sustenance and which is usually central to pleasurable social activities, can pose a constant threat to allergy sufferers.

Food allergy is estimated to affect 11 million Americans, approximately 5 million of whom are children. These children may be allergic to such common foods as eggs, milk, nuts, and seafood. Food allergy occurs when the body's immune system "attacks" otherwise harmless proteins in foods. That assault can cause sudden life-threatening reactions, but it can also result in other debilitating and chronic health problems for children. Food-allergic diseases are sometimes difficult to recognize, but once they have been identified, treatment usually brings significant relief.

The goal of this book is to help you to understand your child's food allergy, which will allow you to

- *recognize symptoms of an allergic reaction;*
- *discuss your concerns with your doctor and your child's caregivers;*
- *understand the results of allergy tests;*
- *explain food allergies to your child; and*
- *keep your child safe.*

In Part 1, I explore how the immune system causes food allergies, including anaphylaxis, a severe allergic reaction. I also consider how food can cause illnesses that may resemble a food allergy but are not. You will see how food allergy can cause or contribute to diseases that affect the skin, gastrointestinal tract, breathing, and even behavior and development. Understanding how allergies occur will help you recognize signs of food allergy and will help you get the most out of the discussions of diagnosis, treatment, and prevention.

1 ~ Food Allergy

The Nuts and Bolts

The immune system is charged with the daunting task of protecting us from a wide range of harmful invaders, such as viruses, bacteria, and parasites. This is no simple endeavor because these germs come in many shapes and sizes and pull all sorts of tricks to evade being found and destroyed by the immune system. To make matters worse, many bacteria are harmless or needed by the body to maintain health, and so the immune system must intelligently ignore certain germs. The challenge to the immune system is complicated because germs may enter the body through a variety of portals. We breathe them in and we eat them, and they get in through irritated or broken skin, such as a cut.

The immune system must be ready to use a variety of approaches to control infection no matter the circumstance. Let's say a few harmful bacteria enter your body during dinner. The immune system must locate and destroy these invaders in a sea of lettuce, tomato, cucumbers, potatoes, beef, carrots, milk, and whatever else might have been in the meal that included the spoiled icing on your cake. Considering that the immune system must simultaneously locate and destroy invaders and ignore "good bacteria" and harmless food proteins, it's no wonder that mistakes are sometimes made. When the immune system attacks harmless food proteins, we suffer food allergies.

To meet these diverse challenges of infection and to destroy invaders, the immune system uses a wide range of strategies. Picture a military operation with land, sea, and air forces; snipers; ground troops; various weapons; "smart bombs"; military leaders who stay at the edge of the fray and troops that venture deep into battle; factories working to make weapons; and so forth, and there you have the immune system—and the makings of big trouble if things go wrong. One way the immune system attacks is to make a protein that can recognize and attach to an invader. This type of protein is called an *immunoglobulin* (im-yoo-no-glob-'yuh-lin) *antibody.*

Immunoglobulin antibodies are programmed to attach to a particular shape or structure on an invader. They are so good at this task that they can make it through all of the muck and "good germs" of a meal and find the "bad germ" to destroy. These immunoglobulins, abbreviated *Ig* (pronounced "eye-gee"), come in a variety of types; each does a different job in attacking germs that have entered the body. For example, *IgG* is a type that is good at attacking germs that float around in the bloodstream, and *IgA* attacks germs on the surface of the gastrointestinal tract or the breathing passages. It is the antibody called *IgE* that causes the most trouble with allergy.

IgE, the Focus of Trouble

IgE is special. Not only does it float around in the bloodstream, but it also attaches itself to certain cells that the immune system uses to fight germs, enabling these otherwise ignorant cells to detect specific invaders. Imagine IgE as an antenna that can only see one particular signal. Thousands of IgE antibodies stud the surface of immune system worker cells called *mast cells* and *basophils,* allowing these cells to "see" whatever the IgE antibody "antennae" can detect. Mast cells reside in the respiratory tract, intestines, skin, and other body organs, and basophils float in the bloodstream. Mast cells and basophils are preloaded with chemicals such as histamine that they can release if the IgE antibodies detect a signal. Researchers believe this system was originally designed to fight parasite infections, and so parasites are one possible "signal" that could be detected. For example, a worm might enter the body, or travel within the body, and come in contact with these armed mast cells and basophils. The IgE antennae would attach to the parasite, alerting the cell to release its load of chemicals immediately to destroy the parasite. Additional chemicals released from the mast cells and basophils alert other members of the immune system of the trouble, tantamount to a radio signal calling in the troops. The successful battle ends with the death of the parasite.

But what if the system becomes misdirected? What if those IgE antibodies recognize harmless proteins in pollens, animal danders, or foods? In these circumstances, the "E" in IgE should stand for "Evil" because this is the root of the problem with allergy, including food allergy (other examples are hay fever, asthma, and bee sting allergy). The IgE antibodies are primarily directed toward proteins, so it is helpful to understand what a protein is, and how a protein is different from other components of foods.

Food is a complex mixture of fats, sugars, carbohydrates, other nutrients, and proteins. Cow's milk, for example, comprises milk fat, milk sugar (called *lactose*), various minerals and nutrients, and more than twenty different proteins. Two types of common milk proteins are casein and whey. Proteins comprise long chains of molecules called *amino acids.* Amino acids are like beads on a baby bracelet. Imagine a long baby bracelet with beads that spell out the sentence: "This is a cow's milk protein." The IgE antibody may be directed to a particular segment of this sentence such as "a cow's" or "milk pro." It is also possible, because these proteins are scrunched up and folded (like scrunching the bracelet in the palm of your hand), that the IgE will see the words "This . . milk" next to each other in the folded bracelet. When the IgE antibodies specific to that spot on the particular milk protein attaches, the mast cell is alerted and releases chemicals like histamine that produce symptoms such as itchy rashes or worse.

Maybe your child is allergic to cats, oak tree pollen, and peanuts. IgE antibodies—little antennae that recognize proteins from these three triggers—are made by special cells of the immune system called "B cells." The IgE antibodies float in the bloodstream and enter various areas of the body as they find their way to mast cells in the skin, nose, lungs, and gastrointestinal tract. Now the mast cells, studded with little "cupholders" that grip the tail of these IgE antennae, become armed with a mixture of antennae that can grab protein from cat, oak, or peanut. Without exposure to these proteins, all is quiet. But what happens when your child visits a friend's home where two cats live, and the cat dander proteins hit her nose and eyes? Trouble begins as the IgE studding the surfaces of mast cells in those body locations detects cat dander proteins. Even though the mast cell is armed against peanut, oak, and cat, the cat dander IgE antibodies will attach, and the mast cells in the nose and eyes will spew histamine, a release of histamine leads to sneezing; red, itchy, watery eyes; and a lot of discomfort. Taking an *anti*histamine medication and leaving the friend's home provides relief. Being at a friend's home with dogs does not affect your child because your child has not made IgE antibodies to dog dander proteins (which look different to the immune system than cat protein).

If your child ate peanuts, the problem could be worse. Once the peanut protein is absorbed during digestion, it enters the bloodstream and finds its way to peanut-detecting IgE antibodies on mast cells in various areas such as the skin (possibly causing hives), respiratory tract (asthma symptoms), intestines (vomiting and diarrhea), and possibly the circulatory system. Unlike the reaction when the cat protein simply touched the eyes and nose, the reaction when large numbers of mast cells are activated in this way from peanut protein may result in a rapid release of tremendous amounts of chemicals leading to severe allergic reactions. This is when the real trouble begins: a life-threatening food allergy. Food-allergic reactions that depend on the IgE antibodies, whether the reactions are severe or mild, are called *IgE-mediated food allergies.*

As you can imagine, it was not supposed to happen this way. The immune system is designed to protect, not hurt, us. Many people mistakenly assume that allergy develops from a weak immune system. In fact, allergy and food allergy represent a strong, but misdirected, immune response. In later chapters, we will see how measuring this aberrant immune response can be used to diagnose food allergies, how medications can interrupt the responses to reverse symptoms, and what research advances have been made toward treating, preventing, and, we hope, curing food allergies. We will also explore why our current living environment has led so many of us and our children to experience food and other allergies. But first, let's take a look at how the immune system can cause food allergy in ways other than through "IgE-vil" antibodies and that foods can make your child sick in ways that may look like, but are not, food allergies.

The Immune System Attacks Foods in Other Ways, Too

The immune system is not a "one trick pony" and must fight invaders in many ways other than through Ig. Indeed, a variety of cells and various chemical messengers protect us from infection. One such cell is called a *T cell.* This is the army general of the immune system, calling in specific troops for particular battles. The available arsenal is diverse, but in regard to allergy, the T cell releases signals that call on a type of immune cell called the *eosinophil* (e′ə-sin′ə-fil). Huge collections of eosinophils characterize allergic inflammation (swelling), and inflammation is the main feature of chronic allergic diseases such as asthma, hay fever, persistent allergic skin rashes (eczema or atopic dermatitis), and certain chronic gastrointestinal diseases. It is thought that the eosinophil, like mast cells and IgE, is important in the battle against parasites. The eosinophils arrive at sites of the body where the T cells have alerted them to trouble. When they get there, they release chemicals that lead to swelling, itching, and irritation.

If the T cell "generals" have decided that a food protein is an enemy, they may employ one of three strategies: (1) tell B cells to make IgE antibodies (causing IgE-mediated reactions); (2) tell eosinophils to come to locations where the food proteins have been detected by these T cells; or (3) activate both parts of the immune response. When the T cells direct allergic inflammation that does not involve IgE antibodies, allergists call this a *non-IgE-mediated food allergy.* If both arms of the immune system are activated, this is called a *mixed IgE and non-IgE response.* These types of immune system attacks on food proteins affect health in several ways. Children may experience severe and chronic skin rashes that interrupt sleep and affect social interactions and may even impede growth. Infants and children may experience symptoms of indigestion (reflux), vomiting, diarrhea, and poor growth because a food allergy is affecting the intestines. The problems caused by mixed or non-IgE antibody food allergies are significant but can be corrected once the problem foods are identified and eliminated from the child's diet.

In Chapters 2, 3, and 4, we explore the symptoms and disorders of non-IgE-related food allergies. Diagnosing this type of food allergy is complicated because simple allergy tests to detect the IgE antibody antennae, which is relevant to sudden food-allergic reactions, are typically irrelevant when exploring the role of foods in these chronic diseases. The diagnosis of chronic problems (intestinal, skin, breathing) is also complicated because they can be triggered by allergens other than foods.

Your doctor must consider a variety of explanations when faced with a particular illness. In the case of food allergy, a major question arises: Is this an allergy to foods that involves IgE antibodies? But another vital question is: If this illness is related to a food, is it a food allergy (an immune response to a food protein) or is it another type of adverse reaction to a food?

When Adverse Reactions to Foods Are Not Allergies

Wayne, a healthy 4-year-old, was brought to see me by his parents who were worried about a food allergy. He developed a bright red rash on separate occasions within minutes of eating strawberries, cinnamon gum, lemon-drop candies, corn chips with salsa, and ten other foods. Wayne's parents brought along blood test results that his pediatrician had done. Although the blood tests were performed to a large range of foods, they failed to show evidence of an allergy. The family was concerned that future reactions might be quite severe and did not understand why tests to various foods were negative. In the meantime, they were severely restricting Wayne's diet.

When a possible food allergy is evaluated, the first step is to take a careful history to determine whether the illness fits the description of an immune response to a food. Other potential diagnoses include an adverse reaction to foods which is not an immune response and illnesses having nothing to do with foods. In Wayne's case, I was interested not in the tests performed for allergy but in his symptoms. The medical history revealed that the rash always developed along his right cheek, which was not itchy or swollen, that the rash only occurred while he was eating and lasted only a few minutes, and that he had no other symptoms. In addition, the foods associated with the reaction appeared to have little in common. It was clear that the response was food related, but was this an allergy? Many features of allergy were missing: no itch, no other symptoms. And why was the "rash" always on the right cheek?

I explained to Wayne's family that there was no need for more testing, and no need to fear the foods. Wayne had a disorder called *gustatory flushing syndrome.* Foods that made him salivate heavily, such as tart and spicy foods, activated a nerve in his cheek that caused blood vessels to dilate leading to a "blush." The disorder is not dangerous and often resolves with time. Wayne's adverse reaction to a food was not a food allergy because the immune system was not involved. Wayne could safely resume a normal diet.

A food can cause illness in many ways without involving the immune system. Food poisoning is an obvious example. Nearly anyone who eats spoiled food will experience illness, usually gastrointestinal symptoms. One type of food poisoning can actually mimic food-allergic reactions. There was a case in the early 1990s, at a well-known hotel in New York, in which a number of lawyers experienced symptoms that included an itchy mouth, hives, face redness, and vomiting after eating tuna. Of course, these symptoms match the description of a food-allergic reaction, but what is the likelihood that several adults simultaneously developed an allergy to tuna fish? A type of food poisoning called *scombroid fish poisoning* caused the reaction. When dark-meat fish, such as tuna or mahi-mahi, spoils, histamine-like chemicals are formed in the fish and can cause what appears to be an allergic reaction when ingested. In this instance, a food allergy was not to blame, which was fortunate for the lawyers but not for the hotel!

Recall that food allergy represents an immune system assault on food *proteins.* Therefore, other food components, namely, fats, sugars, vitamins, minerals, and chemical constituents, including nonprotein coloring additives and preservatives, would not typically be expected to cause an allergic response. That is not to say that these other components are unable to cause other types of adverse effects.

Certain nonimmune adverse reactions to foods are simply a predictable response to irritant chemicals or pharmacologic (druglike) components in food. You have likely teared up while cutting onions—an expected reaction. I typically drink one or two caffeinated beverages each day. For me, this is medicinal because if I don't have these drinks, I develop a headache and feel drowsy. However, if I drink four or five caffeinated beverages a day, I sweat, shake, and have heart palpitations. I am not "allergic" to caffeine, but to some degree, I succumb to its pharmacologic, or drug, effects. Similarly, orange vegetables contain carotene, a yellow-orange pigment. Infants who eat primarily yellow squash and carrots will often develop a yellow-orange skin glow from these foods, an expected outcome of ingesting this nutrient.

Some pharmacologic effects of food components are less predictable and depend much on the individual's level of sensitivity to them. Some people are more sensitive to caffeine's adverse effects, and they experience palpitations after consuming small amounts. Persons with migraine headaches sometimes notice that certain foods, such as hard cheeses, wine, and fermented foods, trigger their headaches. Some individuals are particularly sensitive to capsaicin, the chemical that makes spicy food "hot." They have hay fever symptoms when eating such foods because capsaicin activates nerves leading to a sneeze reflex and runny nose. Anyone who has accidentally sniffed black pepper has also experienced this reaction.

Many adverse reactions to foods occur because an individual has an *intolerance* to a component of the food. In most cases, a weakened or absent ability to digest a sugar causes the intolerance. Lactose intolerance is a classic example. A person who is unable to digest the milk sugar lactose, a problem often due to an inherited deficiency in the digestive enzyme lactase, may experience symptoms such as diarrhea and stomach upset. The degree of discomfort depends on the amount of milk sugar consumed. For young children, lactose intolerance is often a short-lived problem that occurs following a stomach virus. A stomach virus may temporarily damage the intestinal lining where the lactase enzyme usually resides. Once recovered, the lining is able to digest the lactose again. This is why your pediatrician may advise you to avoid milk and milk products for a number of days after this type of illness.

The types and amounts of fats, fiber, and sugars in your child's diet could cause various changes in your child's stool. Often, changes in stool frequency or consistency lead parents to suspect a food allergy. In fact, many of the diet-related changes in stool pattern are predictable and are not the result of any illness. For example, many beans contain a sugar called saffrose that is difficult to digest. Depending on the amount eaten, increased intestinal gas and loose stools can result. Similarly, certain foods contain high amounts of fat, some contain hard to digest particles (corn kernel skins), and others have high concentrations of sugars (fruit juices). Each of these components can cause changes in the stool pattern, or stomach upset, depending on the child and the amount eaten. Dietary changes to reduce discomfort may be recommended by your pediatrician, but these problems attributable to foods are not food allergies.

Most of the time, a physician can diagnose a food intolerance through a careful history. Lactose intolerance may be likely if ingestion of one glass of milk causes an upset stomach and loose stools, while a small amount of butter with much less lactose than the entire serving of milk is tolerated. In some circumstances, lactose tolerance tests, performed by having you consume a lactose-containing drink and then measuring your responses, may be needed for confirmation. Symptoms such as abdominal pain and vomiting and abnormal stool patterns or consistency, usually attributable to foods, can be symptoms of medical disorders unrelated to a particular food. Examples include a variety of diseases that affect the intestines, such as inflammatory bowel disease or cystic fibrosis. You and your physician must keep an open mind: Is this problem attributable to food at all, and if so, is it allergy or another type of adverse food reaction? It is important to discuss your concerns with your doctor. In Chapter 9, we explore how you can help your pediatrician and allergist unravel the cause of your child's symptoms by providing key clues from your own observations.

Food allergy results when the immune system attacks harmless food proteins. This attack can range from sudden, life-threatening allergic reactions to chronic diseases that affect health daily. Unlike food allergy, other adverse food reactions—usually of less consequence for long-term health and less likely to pose imminent danger—are caused by toxins or pharmacologically active components in foods, or by failure to tolerate certain sugars or fats. To help you understand your child's illness, recognize symptoms, and take action to promote health and safety for your food-allergic child, the rest of Part 1 describes the many ways in which food allergies may affect health.

2 ~ Anaphylaxis

At age 2, Natasha had a small taste of peanut, and her lip swelled slightly. Her allergy tests were positive for peanut, which confirmed that she had a peanut allergy. Among the many things I discussed with Natasha's mother was that peanut allergy can be severe. Even though Natasha's reaction had been mild the first time, Natasha could experience a severe allergic reaction to peanut called *anaphylaxis.* Because of the risk of a severe reaction, I provided the family with information and an emergency plan, which included carefully avoiding peanuts, recognizing symptoms of an allergic or anaphylactic reaction, and providing emergency medicine. One of the emergency medications I prescribed was epinephrine, an injection to improve breathing and blood circulation (discussed in Chapter 13).

Natasha's mother called me several months later very upset. Natasha had developed numerous red, raised marks on her skin and was scratching them constantly. This was the first symptom since the peanut allergy diagnosis. Her mother had given Natasha an antihistamine to stop the itch and was keeping the epinephrine on hand. She wanted to know whether she should use the epinephrine. She knew the medication was "lifesaving" but was unsure whether Natasha's symptoms warranted using it, and she was nervous about giving an injection. She remembered that delay in giving epinephrine had meant death for some people with food allergy and panic was setting in. Was Natasha experiencing anaphylaxis?

Defining Anaphylaxis

When we talk about anaphylaxis (an′ə-f ə-lak′sis), we usually mean "a severe allergic reaction." Scientists often define anaphylaxis as a type of allergic reaction in which IgE antibodies (allergic antibodies) are involved and symptoms occur in parts of the body that have not actually contacted the food. For example, if eating peanuts makes your mouth itchy, or if rubbing peanut on your skin makes the skin red and swollen, that would *not* be considered anaphylaxis because the reaction occurred directly where the peanut touched, not elsewhere on the body.

A few itchy spots on a toe after eating peanuts is not anaphylaxis because everyone would agree this is not a severe allergic reaction. Properly defining and recognizing anaphylaxis should affect treatment decisions. Natasha's mother is not concerned with semantics arguments; she wants to know whether her child needs emergency treatment with epinephrine (ep′ə-nef-rin), a drug that reverses life-threatening symptoms that occur during a severe allergic reaction.

Right now, Natasha has an itchy skin rash called *hives.* Hives, which doctors call *urticaria,* may look like mosquito bites with little raised centers and a ring of redness around them, or they may sometimes meld together in various formations with raised areas and redness. Hives are very itchy. An allergic reaction often includes hives but not always. Hives are often the first symptom of a potentially more severe allergic reaction, but many times they go away with no other symptoms. Hives unrelated to allergies can also occur.

I calmed Natasha's mother and discovered that Natasha had been experiencing a fever and runny nose for a few days. Natasha had almost certainly not eaten anything likely to have contained peanuts. Natasha's mother suspected that peanut allergy may have caused this reaction because Natasha had never before experienced hives like this, and the previous afternoon, Natasha had eaten her grandmother's homemade, supposedly peanut-free, cake. Armed with this additional information about her fever and nasal symptoms, I felt comfortable explaining that Natasha was most likely experiencing a rash due to a virus. It was unlikely that the cake contained peanut. If it did, I would have expected a reaction soon after it was eaten, not a day later. I suggested she take Natasha to her pediatrician for additional evaluation of what was likely to be a viral illness.

Natasha's mother was right to think about food allergy when she saw Natasha's hives. After all, Natasha has a peanut allergy, and hives are a common symptom of an allergic reaction. Although no harm would have been done if Natasha's mother had administered the epinephrine, this circumstance did not require it. In different circumstances, I would have suggested immediate administration of epinephrine, even though the symptom was the same. For example, if Natasha had actually eaten peanut and peanut had previously caused a severe reaction for her, then giving the epinephrine would have been appropriate, even though hives were the only symptom.

It is important for you, your child, and your child's caretakers to know what symptoms can occur during an allergic reaction. Some of these symptoms are dangerous and require emergency treatment with epinephrine, while others may be mild and treatment may depend on your child's past reactions, medical history, and other circumstances during a reaction.

Symptoms of a Food-Allergic Reaction and Anaphylaxis

During a food-allergic reaction, the most common part of the body affected is the skin. Hives, like Natasha experienced, are the most common skin symptom. The skin may also become swollen, a symptom called *edema* (i-dé-mə). Lips and eyelids may swell. The skin can become itchy and red, and sometimes a dry, red, bumpy rash called *eczema,* or *atopic dermatitis,* develops.

The gastrointestinal tract is the next most likely affected system, with symptoms such as an itchy mouth, stomachache, nausea, vomiting, diarrhea, and sometimes an odd, perhaps metallic, taste in the mouth. A person may have cramps either from the stomach or, for postpubertal girls, from uterine contractions. The symptoms described thus far are not intrinsically dangerous.

The danger begins when the respiratory tract or blood circulation is affected, although not every symptom in these parts of the body is necessarily severe. For example, a sudden stuffy and runny nose may signal involvement of the respiratory system. More troubling symptoms include mild coughing or throat clearing. Although these symptoms may simply reflect a child's response to an itch in the nose, mouth, or throat, similar symptoms could occur if the throat is swelling closed. Obvious and potentially dangerous breathing symptoms that may occur if the throat or windpipe is closing include hoarseness, difficulty swallowing, high-pitched honking sounds with breathing, or struggling to breathe. When a child is having trouble breathing, he or she may breathe faster to get more oxygen but may have trouble doing so. The chest may pull in with each breath and the nostrils flare like a rabbit's or horse's nose. Other breathing symptoms include wheezing, a whistling sound from the lungs, and repetitive coughing. In the throes of a breathing problem, the skin may look flushed, but if not enough oxygen is getting in, the skin or lips may turn blue.

If blood circulation is affected a child may become pale and dizzy or even faint. The pulse may be weak, and usually the heart is beating rapidly or, sometimes, slowly. A feeling of impending doom may be described even before symptoms progress. For instance, a child may say that she feels something very bad is going to happen.

During any particular food-allergic reaction, exact symptoms and their order of appearance can vary. One of my patients, 7-year-old Erin, had four allergic reactions to two different foods, egg and peanut, over a two-year period. Her first reaction to egg began with vomiting followed by hives. Her next reaction, to peanut, was severe, with no hives but with stomach pain, coughing, wheezing, and throat tightness. Another ingestion of egg caused hives. During her most recent reaction to peanut, she developed an itchy mouth and a few hives around the lips. The lesson: allergic reactions can vary from time to time.

Mild symptoms that do not affect increasing areas of the body are usually not considered life-threatening anaphylaxis (for example, only a skin rash or only an itchy mouth). When breathing or blood circulation is affected, the allergic reaction is life-threatening anaphylaxis. *Anaphylactic shock* describes a severe allergic reaction when circulation is impaired and blood does not bring nutrients and oxygen to vital organs. Usually, the pulse weakens, and the child may lose consciousness or become disoriented because of poor blood flow to the brain. The heart may beat faster to try to circulate blood, but the blood vessels—tubes that channel blood around the body—become floppy and widen from all the chemicals released during a severe allergic reaction. When the blood vessels are loose and floppy, the blood pools and does not circulate well, and the blood pressure falls.

To recognize a food-allergic reaction in your child and to respond with appropriate treatments, consider both the symptoms of an allergic reaction that are not harmful, although they may be uncomfortable, as well as the symptoms that are already, or may soon become, life threatening.

Examples of Symptoms of an Allergic Reaction That
Are Not Intrinsically Life Threatening

Breathing	Nasal congestion Runny nose (rhinitis) Occasional cough
Gastrointestinal	Nausea Vomiting Diarrhea

	Abdominal pain Itchy mouth/ear canal Lip swelling Odd taste in mouth
Skin	Flushing/red skin Itch Hives Skin swelling Eczema flare
Other	Red/itchy eye Uterine contractions

Each symptom in the following list *by itself may indicate a more life-threatening symptom* that could already reflect impaired breathing or circulation or may be an early sign that breathing or circulation may become compromised.

Examples of Symptoms of an Allergic Reaction That Are or May Soon Become Life Threatening

Respiratory	Throat tightness Wheezing Shortness of breath Repetitive coughing Trouble breathing High-pitched noises when air goes in and out Change in voice/hoarseness Turning pale/blue
Gastrointestinal	Obstructive tongue swelling Trouble swallowing
Cardiovascular	Low-blood pressure (hypotension) Fainting, passing out, losing consciousness Chest pain Dizzy/lightheaded Weak pulse
Other	Feeling of "impending doom"

If your child ingested a food allergen, then the symptoms in the first list may alert you that a food-allergic reaction is occurring; you would then carefully check for worsening symptoms while considering treatment with emergency medications such as epinephrine, an injection to improve breathing and blood circulation. If symptoms from the second list are present, then treatment with epinephrine is needed.

An allergic reaction is scary; however, understanding the symptoms will allow you to recognize a reaction and promptly help your child. Knowing the symptoms can save a life. Failure to recognize a food-allergic reaction, or delays in treatment after a child has had significant symptoms, can be fatal. Proper treatment also means understanding that there are other reasons for some of the same symptoms of allergic reactions to foods, and that specific circumstances during a reaction may help you decide whether anaphylaxis is present or is likely to develop.

Learning to Recognize Anaphylaxis

Jimmy is a 7-year-old with asthma and a severe fish allergy. He brought his own lunch to his friend Eric's home, along with his asthma inhaler and emergency medications, an antihistamine and epinephrine. Jimmy's mother instructed Eric's mother about Jimmy's allergies and also mentioned that Jimmy had a slight "cold" for the past few days. Jimmy knew not to share food with other children to reduce the risk of eating fish. After lunch, he was running outside with his friend and began to cough. When the boys came back inside, Jimmy was coughing repetitively and wheezing. Was Jimmy experiencing anaphylaxis? Wheezing is a serious symptom if this is a food-allergic reaction. Should Jimmy receive treatment for anaphylaxis, an injection of epinephrine?

Many of the symptoms that occur in an allergic reaction can have other causes. A virus or insect bites can cause a hivelike rash. Eczema can flare from a change in weather. Typical allergic symptoms such as wheezing, itchy eyes, and a runny nose could be caused by allergens other than food such as from exposure to cats or pollen. Of course, symptoms that overlap with the symptoms of a food-allergic reaction can be confusing, but it is usually not too difficult to figure out whether a food-allergic reaction is likely if one considers the circumstances. Was there a known or possible exposure to the food? Is there an alternative explanation for symptoms?

Jimmy ate his "safe" lunch and did not eat any unsafe food. Exposure to fish was not a factor but exercising was. Jimmy has asthma and had a runny nose that day. A respiratory virus as well as exercise are common triggers for asthma. A combination of a cold and running around with Eric triggered an asthma "attack." He would benefit from treatment with his asthma inhaler. Jimmy likely was not having a food-allergic reaction.

Symptoms of many different medical problems can mimic symptoms of a food-allergic reaction. Choking can result in coughing or difficulty breathing; mosquito bites may resemble hives; a sore throat may cause swallowing discomfort; distaste for a food may be interpreted as a reaction; symptoms in the gastrointestinal tract such as stomachache, nausea, vomiting, or diarrhea could be caused by a virus but mimic a food reaction; and a "panic attack" with sweating, heavy breathing, and faintness can mimic anaphylaxis.

Many families are concerned that they won't be able to tell which symptoms are from a food-allergic reaction and may overtreat or undertreat their children. However, once I have reviewed with my patients the typical symptoms and circumstances of food-allergic reactions, symptoms that mimic reactions, and allergic problems that can arise apart from foods, I rarely see anyone mistake a food-allergic reaction for some other malady or vice versa. If you are uncertain whether a particular circumstance is a food-allergic reaction, you should give your child the emergency medications anyway. The side effects of the medications are minimal, compared with not treating a severe reaction.

In most situations, it is clear that a food has been ingested and has triggered a reaction. The question then becomes, Is this reaction anaphylaxis? Four-year-old Jenny has a milk allergy. She ate her brother's ice cream, and you notice she has a few hives on her face. Otherwise, she seems fine. Should Jenny be treated for anaphylaxis? Most people might say "no" because Jenny has mild symptoms. Identification of anaphylaxis requires considering not only specific symptoms but also circumstances, including exposure to the food, and the specific allergic history of the child. Right now, you do not know much about Jenny, except that she has a milk allergy. If I told you that Jenny had already experienced four milk-allergic reactions and never had more than hives, you might attribute her current hives to another allergic reaction, not anaphylaxis. But what if Jenny turned pale, cleared her throat, coughed, and vomited? You would probably agree that she needed treatment, namely, epinephrine, for anaphylaxis because multiple areas of her body were affected and there were symptoms of a severe reaction.

Now suppose we return to the beginning: Jenny has a milk allergy and ate her brother's ice cream, but there were no symptoms. Would you give Jenny epinephrine for anaphylaxis? Of course not, because she has no symptoms. But what if she'd had severe reactions to milk four times in the past and was hospitalized for two of those reactions, receiving medications to improve her breathing and promote circulation? You'd agree that with a history of such severe reactions and knowing she ingested milk, treating her for anaphylaxis with epinephrine is a good decision, even though she had no symptoms yet.

To determine whether an allergic reaction is currently anaphylaxis or is likely to become anaphylaxis, you'll require some background information and need to make a few judgments. The judgment usually focuses on three points:

1. Whether ingestion of the problem food was likely
2. The severity of previous reactions
3. The current symptoms

An anaphylactic reaction can be evident apart from any history: if a child rapidly develops typical skin symptom, say, hives *and* severe breathing symptoms (wheezing or trouble breathing or typical circulatory symptoms), then anaphylaxis is likely. But anaphylaxis may also be highly likely if a food allergy is known, a problem food has probably been ingested, and certain symptoms arise soon after. Following ingestion of an allergen, anaphylaxis could be defined by any sign of poor circulation or by *two or more* of the following symptoms or features:

1. Skin involvement (e.g., hives, generalized itch/flush, swollen lips, tongue)
2. Airway compromise (e.g., trouble breathing, wheeze)
3. Gastrointestinal symptoms (e.g., crampy abdominal pain, vomiting)

Even this scheme may not always identify anaphylaxis. A person without a history of a prior severe reaction may have trouble breathing, with asthma and throat tightness, after eating a food and warrant treatment for anaphylaxis. If the listed symptoms and features do occur, the chance a person is experiencing anaphylaxis is high.

Someone with very severe past reactions—such as blood circulation problems like Jenny's—should be treated for anaphylaxis before symptoms occur if the person eats a food that had previously caused a severe reaction. If Jenny had eaten a food and it was unclear whether it contained milk, we might wait to see whether any symptoms develop and, if so, treat for anaphylaxis. If you are ever unsure about the symptoms, however, it is safer to treat for anaphylaxis.

We have seen that recognizing when allergy symptoms are, or may lead to, anaphylaxis requires thought about the circumstances at the time of the reaction, the symptoms observed, any clues available from previous reactions, and consideration of alternative explanations for certain symptoms. In later chapters, we consider the types of medications available, and how you can teach your child and caretakers what they need to know to keep your child safe. We are now ready to consider more about assessing your child's risk of food anaphylaxis.

The Course of Anaphylaxis and Assessing Risks

Baby Elinor was breast-fed and did well, except for mild eczema rashes, until age 10 months when she was given yogurt, her first milk product. Minutes after eating the yogurt, she developed numerous hives all over her body and was treated with an antihistamine. Elinor had already eaten many other foods with no problem, including soy, fruits, vegetables, wheat crackers, and foods containing a small amount of milk, such as bread with a little butter. An allergy blood test confirmed a milk allergy and was also positive for egg and peanut, foods she had not yet eaten. Elinor's parents were rightfully concerned and anxious and came to my office with a long list of questions: How much milk will cause a reaction? Is she allergic to touching or smelling these foods? Will any of her allergies be life threatening? Will her symptoms worsen over time? Will she develop more allergies and will any go away? Will she be OK?

The diagnosis of a food allergy, and possible severe food allergy, provokes anxieties. I had so much to tell Elinor's parents. Most of what I explained would be comforting, but some information would add to their fear and concern. I was able to provide them with general information about the potential for a severe allergic reaction. The information comes from numerous research studies and reports about food-induced anaphylaxis.

The Causal Foods

About 90 percent of food allergies in infants and children are attributable to a small group of foods or food categories: cow's milk, egg, peanut (a food in the bean, or legume, family), tree nuts (e.g., walnut, cashew, pistachio, pecan, Brazil nut, almond, and hazel), soy, wheat, and seafood, such as finned fish (tuna, salmon, cod) and shellfish (shrimp, crab, lobster). It is possible, however, to be allergic to any food. Peanuts, tree nuts, and seafood are the most common offenders for severe and life-threatening anaphylaxis. Next are seeds (sesame), eggs, and milk. Again, any food, even grains (wheat), meats (beef and chicken), fruits, and vegetables could cause anaphylaxis. Given that Elinor had already eaten a variety of foods, the main concern would be for her to avoid common offenders she had not yet tried, foods she had reacted to, and foods for which she tested positive. At her age, many of these foods, for example, nuts, were off-limits because she could choke on them. We would need to monitor her progress over time to determine which foods to add to her diet.

The Risks for Other Allergies and Allergic Diseases

Numerous triggers besides food can cause anaphylaxis and allergic reactions. Elinor's exposure to milk caused hives, but additional common triggers include medications and insect stings. Less common causes are vaccines, latex, allergy treatment shots, and exercise. Sometimes people experience anaphylaxis and no cause is identified, which is called *idiopathic anaphylaxis. Food-associated, exercise-induced anaphylaxis* may occur when exercise follows the ingestion of a particular food to which IgE-mediated sensitivity is usually demonstrable (celery or wheat are common offenders) or, less commonly, after the ingestion of any food. People with this illness are able to eat the food without symptoms and are able to exercise without symptoms if they have not ingested the food in the several hours preceding the physical activity.

Elinor seems to be a child disposed to allergic problems. She had already experienced mild allergic skin rashes—the milk-allergic reaction that brought her to my office—and she tested positive for allergy to several foods. Both of her parents had allergic problems, hay fever, and mild asthma, and these allergic conditions run in families and often occur together. Although it was unlikely Elinor would experience all or even many of the allergic problems (bee sting, drug or latex allergy, exercise anaphylaxis, etc.), she had certain increased risks for allergic problems, and so I had specific advice. Her parents and her doctors would keep an eye out for signs of asthma (wheezing, prolonged cough). She could be treated promptly for this problem if it occurred. Because of a possible egg allergy, she may need to be evaluated to ensure that certain egg-containing vaccines are withheld or given under my supervision. The MMR (measles-mumps-rubella) vaccine is not considered to be a particular risk for a child with egg allergy. However, the yearly influenza vaccine may contain egg, as does the yellow fever vaccine (used for travel to some countries). Therefore, she would require more evaluations before receiving these two vaccines (see Part 4).

The Risks from Various Casual Air or Skin Exposures to Food Allergens

Elinor's parents were particularly nervous about her exposure to milk because milk is so common in many foods, and they had read that some people react to smelling or touching peanut. Would Elinor have anaphylaxis from touching or smelling these foods?

Casual exposure to food allergens from skin contact or by smell is probably one of the most worrisome notions, engendering much more stress than is truly warranted. Part of the reason for the fear may be that the rare cases of reactions from minute exposures or from unusual contact are publicized and emphasized the most because of their dramatic nature. What should perhaps be emphasized is that the vast majority of people with severe, life-threatening food allergies live day to day around the foods they avoid, and as long as they do not eat them, they are fine. Most research studies and clinical experience show that severe reactions occur from ingestion and not from skin contact or breathing fumes.

In a study my colleagues and I conducted, thirty children with severe peanut allergy had a small amount of peanut butter rubbed on the skin for one minute. None had a reaction beyond the point of skin contact with the peanut butter. This is the most likely reaction from skin contact—a reaction on the skin where the food touched and not beyond. We see this most commonly when an individual eats a given food and then kisses a child with an allergy to that food on the cheek. Redness develops at the location of the kiss and typically nothing more. Of course, passionate kissing could transfer food, leading to ingestion and a reaction. Many of my patients experience a rash on their legs when they are wearing shorts and are dining in restaurants. This occurs from skin contact with the residue on seats and highchairs and can be avoided by using a wet wipe on these surfaces. The eye is an area of increased sensitivity. If Elinor had milk residue on her finger and rubbed her eye, redness and dramatic swelling of the eyelids are possible. I would not expect any reactions beyond the eye in this situation, but swollen eyelids can look troubling.

Reactions from inhalation can depend on specific foods and specific situations that lead to high concentrations of airborne food protein. Protein may become airborne as foods heat during cooking. For example, reactions may result when someone is close to rapidly boiling milk, steam from eggs frying, or steam from hot fish. Airborne seafood proteins can cause reactions in seafood markets. In these situations, most reactions to airborne food proteins are similar to a cat-allergic individual's contact with a cat. Symptoms may be hay fever—like itchy eyes and nose and runny nose or an asthmatic response, if the allergic individual has asthma, unlike in severe anaphylaxis when blood pressure can drop. Airborne peanut proteins near peanut butter are harder to detect. My research group had thirty highly peanut-allergic children sniff peanut butter for ten minutes and none reacted. We only tested peanut butter; exposure to a less oily form of peanut, say, peanut flour, that may become airborne could more likely elicit a nasal or breathing reaction.

Although I was not too concerned about Elinor having a reaction from food odor, skin contact leading to ingestion at her age posed a special problem. As an infant, Elinor is likely to place objects in her mouth, and reactions could be more significant. I discussed with her parents the implications for avoiding certain settings, which are reviewed in Part 4.

Amount of Food That Causes a Reaction

The amount of food needed to trigger a reaction can vary. Small contamination levels of food can trigger a reaction in some highly sensitive persons (not a risk that is predictable from allergy tests). Indeed, severe reactions have occurred from trace amounts, such as in cross-contamination in food. However, many persons do not react until higher amounts are ingested. When allergists perform oral food challenges to see whether a child has outgrown an allergy, the child eats increasing amounts of the food and stops if any symptoms occur. Sometimes we will not see any reaction until ounces are ingested. Indeed, Elinor had already ingested small amounts of milk with no obvious problem, but a larger amount triggered her mild allergic reaction.

The Time Course of a Reaction

Symptoms almost always start within minutes after an exposure, although a delay of up to an hour or more is possible. In some unusual instances, a few hours may elapse before the symptoms start. Sometimes a reaction will subside and then restart one to three hours later or, sometimes, longer, with even worse symptoms. This type of delayed response following a quiet period is called a *biphasic* reaction, and the more severe the initial symptoms, the more likely there would be a second wave of symptoms. If Elinor experiences anaphylaxis in the future, I would advise her family to inject her with epinephrine and then take her to an emergency room quickly, perhaps by ambulance. Even if she seemed well, I would want her to stay in the emergency department at least four hours without symptoms because of the possible biphasic reaction. If the reaction were particularly severe, staying under medical supervision for longer than four hours may be suggested. In rare circumstances, anaphylaxis could go on for days.

The Nature of Reactions from Time to Time

Many factors determine the severity of a reaction, but the notion that repeated reactions worsen each time is a myth. Repeated reactions may be milder or more severe. Some research shows that reactions in young children (1- and 2-year-olds) are not as severe as in older persons, partly because older children mention throat symptoms that the younger children may not be able to verbalize or that the older children had developed asthma, which is a risk factor for more severe reactions. Factors that might play a role in the severity of a food-allergic reaction include the amount eaten and underlying health (asthma). Asthma is a risk factor for severe reactions even if the asthma is under control; however, experts maintain that keeping asthma under control is important to reduce the risk of breathing problems if a reaction to food occurred.

Additional factors may play a role in whether a reaction occurs, the time course of a reaction, and its severity. For example, the amount of food in the stomach may affect the speed in which the allergen enters the body. Alcohol consumption, the use of aspirin-related medicines (such as ibuprofen but not acetaminophen), and exercise could sometimes enhance reactions. Some children are simply more "sensitive" than others to a food allergen. That is, a smaller amount of food triggers a reaction for some children, and these children may also be at a higher risk for a severe reaction.

Most studies show that allergy tests *do not* predict a reaction's severity. Whether future reactions will be severe or mild is also "unpredictable." Unfortunately, during a reaction, it is impossible to know what to expect.

Elinor's milk reaction was mild, and milk commonly is associated with reactions that are not anaphylaxis. However, anaphylaxis to milk is still a possibility. Elinor also tested positive to peanut, a more potent allergen, and she is at risk of developing asthma. All of these circumstances indicate that she is at risk for anaphylaxis. Therefore, I reviewed an anaphylaxis care plan with her family. Having epinephrine for Elinor is like having a life insurance policy—Elinor is not likely to need the medication, but if she did, I would want it to be available to her.

The Risk of a Fatal Reaction

Research studies have described several features of fatal food-induced anaphylaxis, and several themes emerge. Most often, the victim had a known food allergy. The most common trigger was peanuts, tree nuts, or seafood. In addition, most victims had asthma and did not receive treatment with epinephrine promptly when serious symptoms had occurred. Persons who are more "sensitive" to a food allergen, ones who experience allergic reactions to ingestion of small amounts, may be at higher risk. Unfortunately, teenagers and young adults are at highest risk because they may eat without being cautious about ingredients, they may deny obvious symptoms and thereby avoid seeking treatment, and they may fail to carry or use epinephrine. Another feature of anaphylaxis associated with fatalities is the absence of, or failure to notice, skin symptoms. People expect to see hives, and if they do not, they may not consider anaphylaxis and delay treatment. It is estimated that in the United States more than thirty thousand episodes of food-induced anaphylaxis occur, and there are one hundred to two hundred deaths each year, including all age groups. These numbers are far from comforting, but to put this in perspective, accidental injuries are estimated to cause about fifty-six hundred deaths per year among children in the United States. I explained to Elinor's parents that food-allergy fatalities in her age group are rare, and milk-related deaths are uncommon. However, this assumes caution is taken with her diet and emergency treatments are used in the event of a reaction. I also explained that Elinor will likely "outgrow" her milk allergy with time, and possibly even her allergy to peanut.

After these explanations and other instructions, Elinor's parents seemed more comfortable with understanding and managing her allergies. I indicated to them that this is a stressful problem but one that should not prevent Elinor from doing the things children her age are able to do, except eating the foods to which she is allergic.

Anaphylaxis is a severe, potentially life-threatening allergic reaction. Persons at greatest risk for severe or fatal reactions have asthma and have an allergy to peanut, tree nuts, or seafood. Fatal reactions are associated with a delay in treatment with epinephrine. Teenagers and young adults appear to be at the greatest risk for fatal food-allergic reactions. More details about medication use and food avoidance are reviewed later in the book.

3 ~ Skin Rashes and Eczema

Most food-allergic reactions affect the skin. When a sudden food-allergic reaction occurs, hives may appear, which usually look like mosquito bites and are typically very itchy. Sometimes hives are larger than mosquito bites, and sometimes many hives coalesce into large shapes. The swelling in the center is called a *wheal;* the surrounding red area is called a *flare.* The skin may also become swollen with fluid, which is known as *angioedema.* Body areas that commonly swell include the lips, eyelids, and ears; the skin often becomes itchy during an allergic reaction. Allergy cells in the skin, the mast cells, release chemicals such as histamine that cause blood vessels to expand (causing redness) and leak (releasing fluid that makes the skin swell). The chemicals also trigger nerves to cause an itch sensation.

Chronic skin rashes may be caused, in part, by a food allergy. *Atopic dermatitis,* a type of skin rash, often occurs in persons with allergic problems. The itchy, dry, persistent rash can last for weeks, months, and sometimes years. The rash takes many forms. Sometimes the skin appears to be boiling with deep redness, flakes, cracks, and crusts. In infants, the rash usually appears as red bumps on the face and outer surfaces of the arms and legs but usually not in the diaper area. As children grow up, the rash often moves to the creases of the neck, elbows, wrists, ankles, and knees. The rash can be severe and affect almost every part of the body, although almost never the nose, and the rash may wax and wane in severity over time.

Although skin rashes are a common symptom of food allergy, many other medical problems can cause rashes that resemble allergic rashes. Your doctor, with your help, will need to consider whether your child's rash is food related.

Hives

Barbara, an otherwise healthy 13-year-old, had been experiencing frequent episodes of hives. For several weeks, and for most days of the week, the hives would appear on various parts of her body. Her family showed me photographs of the hives, which looked like typical mosquito bites. They would come and go but disappeared quickly and completely when she took an antihistamine medication. The family came to me with detailed dietary records and suspected that a food dye or preservative might be the culprit.

I reviewed the diet history carefully but had little suspicion that the rash was from a food, food dye, or preservative. When a food allergy triggers hives, the rash typically begins within minutes of the ingestion and does not usually last beyond an hour or so. When someone experiences days of ongoing hives, I usually exclude foods as a trigger, unless the hives occur after meals and snacks. Also, it is not common to suddenly become allergic to foods that were tolerated in the diet, and Barbara had not eaten anything new or unusual. Food dye or preservative allergy is rare. Overall, Barbara's random pattern of hives did not match a food-allergic reaction: she awoke with hives, even before breakfast.

Hives can occur from a variety of triggers. Some triggers are quite unexpected. Some people get hives from exposure to cold or heat or from sweating. Rare individuals experience swelling from vibration, pressure on the skin, or even from touching water. Hives may develop in places where the surface of the skin is rubbed or scratched, a disorder called *dermographism.* Some hives look different from Barbara's and may have a tiny white center with a large surrounding blotch. Heat or sweating often causes this type of hive. Hives are commonly caused by a viral illness. A hivelike rash may result from insect bites and may appear on the legs or other exposed areas. Triggers other than foods, such as medications and airborne allergens, could also cause hives. Barbara's pattern of hives did not fit a food allergy or any of these other explanations.

Medical history and family medical history helps with diagnosing a medical problem. Barbara's family, while not plagued by allergies, had a history of autoimmune disease, which is when the immune system attacks various parts of the body. Barbara's family had skin and thyroid problems from this type of illness. If the body's immune system "attacks" its own mast cells, the mast cells release histamine that cause hives. This seemed likely to be the case with Barbara. Additional tests showed that Barbara had a mild thyroid condition, confirming my suspicion that her hives were caused by autoimmune disease. Treatment required large doses of antihistamine and thyroid medicine.

Jacob was an allergy-prone 2-year-old, who was allergic to eggs and peanuts. He was diagnosed based on prior reactions from eating these foods and positive allergy tests. Otherwise, Jacob was healthy and growing well with no chronic health problems. Jacob's family came to my office because they noticed he had developed two problems around his mouth. First, a slight redness around the edge of his lip, where the skin was dry and cracked. His 5-year-old sister, Ilana, would ask whether Jacob was wearing clown lips. Second, whenever he drank milk or ate ice cream or yogurt, he developed a few small hives around his lips. The family feared he had developed a milk allergy although he had no rashes after he ate cheese.

A few questions revealed that Jacob habitually licked his lips, causing *lip-licking eczema.* He had irritated the skin around his lips with his own saliva, similar to rashes that sometimes occur around infant pacifiers. Because the skin was slightly cracked, milk protein in liquid form could seep into his skin and trigger slight allergic reactions on the skin. A food that is tolerated when eaten can trigger mild allergic reactions when it is in direct contact with the skin, especially if the skin barrier is already irritated.

Mild allergic hives caused by direct food contact with the skin is called *contact urticaria,* or *contact hives.* Contact hives are common in young allergic infants and children who are sloppy eaters. Unlike hives from a typical food allergy, these hives occur only when the food touches the infant's or child's skin; otherwise, the child tolerates eating the food. It may be difficult and confusing for parents to feed the problematic food or foods to their child. Because of the rashes, families may feel unsure that their child can actually tolerate the food. If this is an issue for your child, talk to your doctor to be sure that continuing the food is right for you and your child.

Jacob clearly tolerated eating milk and milk products, even in large quantities. We just needed to get his skin barrier back to normal. Applying petroleum jelly around his lips reduced the lip licking; his skin healed, and small drops of milk no longer caused rashes.

Atopic Dermatitis (Eczema)

Jesse, a 2-year-old with severe atopic dermatitis, was referred to me by his dermatologist. Most of his body was affected by rash. He did not sleep well because of the itching, and many areas of his skin would crack and bleed.

This disruptive discomfort had been going on since he was just 2 months old. The rash sometimes improved after intense treatments but recurred. He was evaluated by several dermatologists and tried skin-care treatments. Some doctors advised infrequent baths, others advised daily or even twice-daily baths, and his skin had been treated with moisturizers, steroid creams, medicated eczema creams, and antihistamines. Still, the rash always returned.

Atopic dermatitis, an inherited illness, is a form of eczema that often occurs in infants and children with an allergic disposition who have relatives with atopic dermatitis or other allergic problems such as asthma, hay fever, or food allergies. The rash typically comes and goes but can be triggered by skin irritants (soap, sweating, clothing that traps moisture or contains detergents), infections, emotions, and allergies. People call atopic dermatitis the "itch that rashes" because the skin is very itchy and constant rubbing feeds the itch and exacerbates the rash. The skin swells with various cells from the immune system that increase the reactions. The skin loses moisture and does not regulate heat and cold well. Medical treatments aim to reverse these problems. Typical care instructions include:

Add moisture: Soaking baths or wet wraps with lukewarm water, moisturizers applied immediately after patting dry following baths.

Remove infections: Baths to remove crusts and bacteria, use of antibiotic ointments or antibiotics by mouth for skin infections.

Reduce irritation: Cotton clothing, clothes rinsed well to remove detergent, mild soaps and shampoos.

Reduce scratching: Fingernails kept short, skin kept moist, use of antihistamines (possibly antihistamines that induce sleep).

Quell the immune response: Use of various steroid creams and ointments and other nonsteroidal medications to reduce inflammation.

Jesse's family was doing all of these things with no success. What about allergy? Various studies, including ones performed by my research colleagues and me, have shown that about 1 in 3 children with moderate to severe atopic dermatitis has a food allergy. Studies have also shown that a relatively short list of foods may account for nearly 90 percent of the problem. The most frequent triggers are milk, egg, peanut, tree nuts, seafood, soy, and wheat. Studies also show that environmental allergens, such as dust mites and animal dander, may increase the rash.

Jesse ate a regular diet, except he had never tried peanuts, tree nuts, or seafood. His father thought that apple made his skin worse; his mother thought that milk and banana worsened his skin, but they had not removed these foods from the diet. Jesse did not like to eat egg and would spit out this food, but he ate egg in a variety of foods such as pancakes, cake, and cookies. The family also had a cat.

I discussed with Jesse's family the process of evaluating food allergy. A few simple tests would need to be performed. I explained that we would need to observe his skin when he avoided certain foods and then observe whether he tolerated the foods or developed a rash from eating them again. Avoiding various foods is risky, for the reasons in the list below, but Jesse was already suffering quite a bit from severe skin rashes. Food allergies would not likely be the only cause of Jesse's rash, but it was worth eliminating suspect food to determine whether the atopic dermatitis could be controlled. By performing a series of allergy tests, removing several foods from his diet based on the test results, and reintroducing them under doctor supervision, we soon established that Jesse had an egg and milk allergy. Banana and apple did not seem to be a problem, nor were several other foods that were a part of his diet. He also tested positive for cat allergy, so the family boarded the cat with a relative. His family cleaned the house to remove cat allergen. With the new diet, Jesse's skin was 75 percent better and required much less care and fewer medications. He still had periods of rash, but overall he was feeling better and sleeping well, and the family was less stressed. The plan was to reevaluate Jesse's food allergies yearly to see whether he was outgrowing any allergies.

Like Jesse's family, Kari's family brought Kari to my office for an evaluation of atopic dermatitis. Kari was 2 years old and had a dry, itchy rash on her elbows and knees. She scratched these rashes but otherwise was healthy and slept well. The family used topical medications on several occasions, and the rash almost completely disappeared but often returned a few days after the medicine stopped. Her family did not like using the medications, but moisturizers alone did not always help. Kari's family hoped that I could identify foods that could be causing the rash so she would not need any medications. The medical history revealed that Kari ate a regular diet for her age, including the common food allergens egg, milk, wheat, and peanut. She had never had a noticeable problem from foods or from exposure to other types of allergens, such as furry pets. Although Kari's family wanted me to test her for food allergies, I was reluctant for several reasons:

- Children with very mild atopic dermatitis are less likely than children with more extensive rash to have a food allergy.
- When children have atopic dermatitis, they often "test positive" to foods, even though many can tolerate the foods without apparent illness or

increase of the atopic dermatitis rash. Therefore, testing without a specific suspicion of a food allergy can be misleading if the rash is only mild.

When foods are removed from the diet, there are inherent risks that should not be overlooked:

—Removing foods from the diet could have nutritional consequences.

—Removing foods may have social consequences.

—When a child tests "positive" on an allergy test for a food he has eaten routinely, and the food is removed from the diet for a long period of time, a sudden and severe reaction can occur sometimes when the food is reintroduced (assuming the allergy was not outgrown).

For these reasons, risks and benefits must be weighed before a decision can be made to remove food from a child's diet to treat a chronic illness. For Jesse, my opinion and the opinion of his family was that trying to control his severe rash by altering his diet was worth the risk and trouble. For Kari, I maintained that risks of dietary restrictions might outweigh any benefit to her mild rash. Kari's family was primarily concerned about side effects of medications. I was able to calm them because the amount of medicine she needed was small and unlikely to carry any significant side effects. It was also likely that her rash would naturally recede as she got older. We decided to defer allergy tests and see how she managed with a good skin care regimen, with plenty of moisturizers but medicated creams used sparingly whenever they were needed. She did well.

Other Food-Related Rashes

Foods can be related to skin rashes in many ways. Irritation probably causes the most common type of food-related rash. For example, acidic citrus foods may irritate the skin of people with sensitive skin and eczema, particularly in infants with atopic dermatitis whose rash flares wherever these acidic foods dribble on the skin. If I pour battery acid on my skin, I would expect a burning rash, so the acidic foods may cause similar problems for dry, chapped skin. The problem usually disappears when the child is no longer such a messy eater.

Sometimes skin contact with foods can cause an itchy, chronic rash that resembles the poison ivy rash and develops a day or two after initial contact with the trigger. Usually, this type of rash, called *contact dermatitis*, occurs as an occupational problem in food handlers. Another uncommon food-related rash may occur in children with celiac disease. *Celiac disease,* a type of immune reaction to gluten, a protein in wheat and certain other grains, causes various digestive problems. If gluten is not removed from the diet, sometimes sufferers develop a blistering rash called *dermatitis herpetiformis.* In Chapter 1, we met Wayne, who experienced a red blotch on his cheek whenever he ate tart foods. This neurologic response, called *gustatory flushing syndrome,* or *auriculotemporal syndrome,* is not dangerous. Similarly, tart or spicy foods may cause skin redness because they trigger skin blood vessels to dilate in some people. This chemical effect is not allergy.

The skin is the most common part of the body to be affected by food allergies. Some rashes, such as hives, develop soon after a food is eaten and generally resolve in minutes to hours. Certain chronic rashes, such as atopic dermatitis, may be partly attributable to food allergies. Your doctor must consider a number of reasons that your child may have a rash. If your child's rash is caused by a food allergy, avoiding the food can result in significant relief.

4 ~ Gastrointestinal Problems

A baby spits up frequently, another infant has bloody diarrhea, a child experiences frequent vomiting and diarrhea and is not growing well, and a teenager has severe "heartburn" and pain when he swallows. What do these individuals have in common? They all may have a food allergy that causes a problem in their digestive system. Or, their symptoms may be caused by something other than food allergy. The gastrointestinal tract tells us when it is sick with just a few symptoms (pain, vomiting, diarrhea, etc.), and there are many reasons it may become sick. For example, the gastrointestinal tract may be affected by infections, digestion problems, ulcers, and numerous other diseases. When an immune reaction to food causes illness, the problem can be called a food allergy and is treatable by removing the causal food allergen from the diet. However, diagnosing food allergy when the only symptoms affect the gastrointestinal tract is tricky because many intestinal problems cause identical symptoms as those presented by a food allergy. Complicating the diagnosis is that when a food allergy causes a gastrointestinal problem, it is often difficult to identify the causal food or foods.

Many disorders can cause problems in the gastrointestinal tract. A doctor will evaluate your child's pattern of illness and consider the most likely culprit. When certain patterns of symptoms occur, and when symptoms develop after certain foods are eaten, then a food allergy is possible and deserves more consideration. The immune system often attacks a food protein using IgE antibodies; however, many of the food allergies that affect the gut occur without these antibodies. Instead, the T cells and other immune cells may cause the trouble.

Bloody Stools in Infants (Proctocolitis)

There are relatively few reasons for infants to have blood in their stools. Your pediatrician will consider whether there is a tear near the anus (called a fissure), an infection, or intestinal obstruction. If there are mucousy, bloody stools without other signs of illness, then this symptom may be attributed to an immune reaction in the colon and rectum. When these symptoms are caused by a food allergy, the disorder is called *allergic proctocolitis,* which typically occurs in breast-fed babies, although sometimes it develops in formula-fed infants. The illness is caused by an immune reaction to cow's milk ingested by the mother and passed through her breast milk. Rarely, other foods such as soy or egg may be to blame. Usually, not much blood is lost, the baby does not become anemic (low blood count), and the bleeding resolves in a day or two after the mother removes or reduces the causal food in her own diet. If the infant is already on a formula, switching to a "hypoallergenic" formula (see Chapter 23) usually stops the bleeding.

If the cause of an infant's bloody stool is unclear, various tests may be needed. If the infant appears generally well but has bloody stools, then a pediatric gastroenterologist might perform a biopsy by placing a small tube in the anus to snatch a bit of the lining of the rectum to determine whether it is healthy. If the illness is allergic proctocolitis, the biopsy will reveal many allergy cells, called *eosinophils,* when viewed under a microscope. With this disorder, infants usually do not appear sick, standard allergy tests (discussed in Chapter 10) are negative, and the problem is usually outgrown by the first year. Breast-feeding can usually be continued with diet restrictions for the mother. For formula, use of a hypoallergenic type should resolve the bleeding (see Chapter 23).

Diarrhea, Poor Growth, and Swelling (Protein Enteropathy)

Although rare, sometimes a food, typically milk, will cause modest swelling or inflammation in an infant's small intestine. If this part of the intestine is affected, sometimes an infant will actually loose nutrients (proteins) into the intestines, leading to poor growth and diarrhea, a food allergy called *enteropathy.* This may be one aspect of other food-allergic disorders (discussed in this chapter) or may occur on its own. An infant with enteropathy may have poor growth, diarrhea, and swelling of the skin (especially the eyelids and legs) because proteins needed to maintain fluid balance are lost in the stools. Many illnesses that can lead to similar symptoms in an infant have nothing to do with food allergies. However, when the inflammation in the small intestine is caused by food, the illness is called *food protein enteropathy.* Avoiding the problem food leads to complete improvement. Like proctocolitis syndrome, the typical allergy tests are negative, and most infants lose the allergy in the first two years. This rare illness is diagnosed by a biopsy showing inflammation in the intestine and by a child's response to eliminating milk or other causal foods from the diet.

Severe Episodic Vomiting, Diarrhea, and Poor Growth in Infants (Enterocolitis; Food Protein–Induced Enterocolitis Syndrome)

Morgan came to my office after experiencing a rather troubling number of illnesses. She had been fed a cow's milk–based infant formula, and by age 2 weeks was spitting up frequently, stopped growing, and had loose stools. Morgan was switched to a soy formula, but within a few days, she was again vomiting and having diarrhea. She was then started on a hypoallergenic formula and did well for two weeks. Morgan's family resumed using a milk-based formula. Two hours after her feeding, Morgan began to vomit repeatedly and appeared quite pale, almost ashen, and weak. She was rushed to the hospital.

Morgan looked blue, was limp, and continued to vomit. She was given intravenous fluids and antibiotics, and her blood tests showed a high white cell count, a sign of infection. Morgan was kept in the hospital to receive antibiotics, but no source of infection could be found. On the second day in the hospital, she was again fed the cow's milk formula. Two hours later, she experienced the same dramatic symptoms. The physicians then realized that her symptoms were not caused by an infection. Her symptoms occurred after she ingested cow's milk and were caused by an allergic reaction to the milk. They fed her the hypoallergenic formula instead, and she did very well.

Morgan had experienced all of the typical symptoms of a food allergy called *food protein–induced enterocolitis syndrome* (FPIES). This is a somewhat rare, but dramatic, form of food allergy that often mimics an infection and is difficult to diagnose unless the problem occurs more than once. The difficulty is that the symptoms closely mimic the symptoms of a gastrointestinal tract infection. The most common FPIES triggers are cow's milk and soy. When a child with FPIES has been consuming the problem food, her intestines become inflamed (swollen with cells from an immune system "attack"), and vomiting, diarrhea, and poor growth may occur. When the child stops ingesting the causal food, all symptoms subside. But the odd part about the disorder is that if the child eats the problem food again, a dramatic onset of vomiting, weakness, sometimes blue skin color, and poor blood circulation occurs after about a two-hour delay. A few hours later, the child may have diarrhea, sometimes with blood in the stool.

The particular symptoms and their severity may vary from time to time or from one child to the next. Treatment involves stopping the food, giving fluids, usually intravenously, and administering steroids, a medication that calms the activity of immune system cells and may help to quell the reaction. T cells (see Chapter 1) may release the chemicals that cause this illness because IgE antibodies only rarely are detected by standard allergy tests. In other words, typical allergy tests are almost always negative with this illness.

Milk is the most common food to cause this dramatic illness. Unfortunately, soy, which is a protein used in soy-based infant formula, is the next most common trigger. If an infant consuming a formula is diagnosed with this problem, a hypoallergenic formula (not soy or milk) should be prescribed. These dramatic symptoms usually do not occur while an infant is breast-feeding. But they can begin once a breast-fed infant starts eating solid foods. In studies performed by me and my colleagues, rice and oat are the most common triggers, with reactions similar to those Morgan experienced.

When an infant develops FPIES to any food, you may be instructed to avoid introducing certain foods that have been associated with these reactions (unless they are already tolerated in the diet). For example, milk, soy, oat, rice, and chicken are the most common offenders, while cooked fruits and vegetables, typically purchased as infant foods in jars, are rarely a problem. Your doctor will likely recommend that your child avoid problem foods until she is older (over 12–18 months) and may recommend introducing certain foods under physician supervision if a reaction is likely.

Standard allergy tests are not relevant to this illness because IgE antibodies detected by the tests are not a cause of this illness. Your allergist may need to do a "food challenge," a medically supervised gradual feeding to determine whether your child is allergic to the foods. When Morgan was 2 years old, I performed this test. During a hospital stay, I fed Morgan milk, which she tolerated. When I fed her soy formula, she developed severe vomiting two hours later and had a low blood pressure. I administered intravenous fluids and steroids for treatment. A year later, I repeated the soy feeding under the same close observation, and she tolerated it. Most children outgrow their FPIES over one to three years, but some may continue to react for many years.

Although there are no reports of deaths from this illness, the reactions are very dramatic and appear to be life threatening. When I make this diagnosis, I instruct families on strict food avoidance and provide an emergency plan as described in Chapter 16. Unlike typical anaphylaxis, treatment of FPIES often requires intravenous fluids and steroids. Because this is a rare, but severe, type of food allergy, I generally provide my patients with a letter that they can take with them to the emergency room that explains the illness. The letter is individualized but includes the following information:

Dear Doctor (To Whom It May Concern),

My child has a food allergy called food protein–induced enterocolitis syndrome. This is a type of allergy that usually does not result in typical "allergic" symptoms such as hives or wheezing but rather in isolated gastrointestinal symptoms.

The foods that my child is avoiding include: ______.

The symptoms of this type of allergic reaction include repetitive vomiting that may not start until a few hours (e.g., 2) following ingestion of the food to which my child is allergic. Even eating trace amounts can trigger a reaction. There is often diarrhea that starts later (after 6 hours). In some cases (about 20%), the reaction includes hypotension and lethargy, sometimes acidemia and methemoglobinemia. The treatment is symptomatic and can include intravenous fluids (e.g., normal saline bolus, hydration) and steroids for significant symptoms. The latter is given because the pathophysiology is that of a T cell response.

This information is being given so that it can be considered in the differential diagnosis for my child in the event of symptoms. Of course, my child having this illness *does not* preclude the possibility of other illnesses (e.g., infection, toxic ingestion) or even other types of allergic reactions leading to symptoms, so it is up to the evaluating physician to consider all possibilities. Similarly, the treating physician is encouraged to pursue any other treatments deemed necessary (e.g., symptomatic such as epinephrine for shock, antibiotics for presumed infection).

Sincerely,
Your Name

This letter is useful because it alerts the doctors to the illness. It describes, in medical terms, some of the typical symptoms such as increased acid in the blood (acidemia), low blood pressure (hypotension), and a blue color (methemoglobinemia) to the skin. The letter also reminds the doctor that there could be other reasons that your child is sick. Of course, if your child has this illness, and you know that your child has ingested the trigger food, you should go to the emergency room for observation.

Allergic Inflammation in the Gastrointestinal Tract (Eosinophilic Esophagitis and Gastroenteritis)

Twelve-year-old Mark was referred to my office following an evaluation by a pediatric gastroenterologist. Mark had had two episodes where food became lodged in his esophagus, which is designed to squeeze food from the mouth down into the stomach. On both occasions, an emergency department doctor used a tube to push the food down into Mark's stomach. During a later evaluation, a biopsy of the esophagus was conducted during an endoscopy. A tube placed into the esophagus, stomach, and other areas of the gastrointestinal tract was used to look at the surfaces of the lining of the digestive tract and to snatch small samples. The gastroenterologist saw that Mark's esophagus did not look healthy. The biopsy found large numbers of eosinophils, a possible sign of allergy.

In my interview with Mark and his family, I discovered that Mark had been experiencing some discomfort with food "going down" for years, but he did not realize this was unusual. He generally chewed his food very well and drank water to alleviate the problem. Mark also had allergies, including hay fever, mild asthma, and a long-standing peanut allergy. As an infant, Mark had an apparent cow's milk allergy that caused vomiting. Considering the symptoms and biopsy findings, it seemed that Mark had an illness called *eosinophilic esophagitis,* a type of allergy that results in allergic cells, eosinophils, collecting in the esophagus. This causes swelling and difficulty in food going down to the stomach. After a variety of allergy tests and trial diets, followed by repeated endoscopies, Mark was kept on a restricted diet and his symptoms eased.

Several types of gastrointestinal allergies result in eosinophils collecting in various parts of the gut. Depending on the amount of inflammation and swelling, symptoms can vary but may include vomiting, pain, loose stools, feeling full after just a small amount of food, poor appetite, and poor growth. In Mark's case, primarily the esophagus was affected, leading to problems with food going to the stomach. This is the most common type of allergic problem related to eosinophils in the gut. Like Mark, affected persons are usually diagnosed in later childhood and early teen years, and they often have other allergic problems.

The eosinophilic gut disorders are named according to the location of the inflammation in the gastrointestinal tract; for example, if many areas are affected it is called *eosinophilic gastroenteritis* (stomach and small intestines). When the small intestine is affected, food is not absorbed well and a child may not grow or gain weight properly. The swelling can be extreme and, rarely, the intestines can become blocked. Persons with these types of eosinophilic gut disorders, whether in the esophagus or other parts of the gastrointestinal tract, usually have relief when the causal foods are identified and removed from the diet. But diagnosis is difficult because typical allergy tests are not very accurate for this illness. It is often hard to know whether the swelling and inflammation have improved without performing invasive tests, such as biopsies. It can take weeks for swelling to improve, and accidental exposure to causal foods can increase symptoms. Because of these difficulties, affected children are often first placed on restricted diets, such as a nonallergenic formula, perhaps applesauce, or a few other foods to see whether diet can control the disease. If this is the case, additional foods are slowly added to the diet.

For some children, the disorder is not food-responsive. For many others, a combination of treatments is needed, such as steroids or other medications to reduce the swelling and quell the immune response, antacid medications to reduce acid irritation, and diet changes to remove possible triggers. Many of these treatments have possible side effects a doctor must carefully monitor. No comprehensive long-term studies on this disorder have been conducted, but it appears that the illness may resolve during infancy, while it may remain a long-lived illness for older children. The primary reason for treatment, besides relief of symptoms, is to reduce inflammation to prevent scarring. Scarring of the esophagus, for example, could result in severe difficulties in food going down into the stomach.

Colicky Infants

Parents may believe their infant has "colic" when the baby frequently cries, has excess gas, and spits up. However, a formal diagnosis of colic involves only crying. An infant has colic if he cries three or more hours a day at least three days each week. Numerous studies have focused on how diet contributes to colic. While some studies show that changing a baby's formula helps, other studies disagree. Colic affects breast-fed infants and formula-fed infants alike. Does colic indicate a food allergy? One assumption is that infants who have other symptoms of cow's milk allergy, such as skin rashes,

IN DEPTH ON EOSINOPHILIC GASTROINTESTINAL DISEASE

Eosinophilic gastrointestinal disease appears to be increasing. The disorder occurs when allergy cells, called eosinophils, collect in the lining of the gastrointestinal tract. Symptoms depend on where in the gut allergy cells have collected to cause the inflammation and the number of cells that have collected, because the more cells there are, the worse the symptoms. When the esophagus is involved, the typical symptoms include pain in the chest when food is traveling down to the stomach and, sometimes, food getting stuck in the esophagus. Additional symptoms resemble heartburn. When allergy cells collect in other parts of the gastrointestinal tract, for example, the stomach or small intestine, different problems may occur such as stomach pain, nausea, and poor appetite. If the small intestine is greatly inflamed, the body loses proteins from the blood into the intestine. When this occurs, the amount of protein in the blood is decreased, which leads to a variety of problems such as fluid imbalances and swelling of the skin (edema) and various body tissues. These problems can also lead to poor growth.

Aside from eosinophilic gastrointestinal disease, other diseases and medical problems can cause pain, swallowing trouble, nausea, vomiting, and swelling. If your physician suspects an eosinophilic gut disease, he would typically order a biopsy to identify these allergy cells or some other explanation for the problems. The biopsy is done during an endoscopy, in which a tube is inserted into the gut through the mouth or nose. This procedure is generally performed by a gastroenterologist while your child is under anesthesia. The doctor can look at the gut lining through the tube to assess the problem and also can snatch bits of the lining of the esophagus, stomach, or intestine—a biopsy—that later can be evaluated under a microscope for allergy cells or other abnormalities. The tube may also be placed up the anus and into the large intestine and rectum to look for problems. Sometimes, other explanations are found for the problem, such as an infection or nonallergic gut disease. Finding large numbers of the eosinophils would suggest an allergy.

Several reasons explain why an allergy is the suspected cause of these eosinophilic gastrointestinal diseases, and why "allergic" is often attached to the identification of eosinophils in the gut. First, the involvement of eosinophils always raises the possibility of allergy because this cell is often seen in diseases with allergic inflammation such as asthma or hay fever. Second, most individuals diagnosed with these problems have other signs of allergic disease, including asthma and environmental allergies to pollens or animal dander, and, very frequently, these individuals have a history of allergic reactions to a variety of foods. In most cases, it is possible to measure the presence of IgE antibodies to various foods. But for some individuals with the same type of inflammation, IgE antibody tests to foods are all negative.

At first, doctors did not think that food allergy was related to finding eosinophils in the gastrointestinal tract. Specifically, when gastroenterologists would find large numbers of eosinophil cells in the esophagus, they often attributed their presence to reflux. Reflux occurs when stomach acid moves up into the esophagus instead of down into the small intestines. This is sometimes thought to happen when a small muscle valve between the esophagus and stomach is somehow weakened and allows stomach juices to seep up and burn the esophagus. The eosinophilic cells that collect after this "burn" were thought to reflect the inflammation and healing resulting from reflux. However, antireflux medications did not always make things better, especially when large numbers of eosinophils were found.

Symptoms for individuals with eosinophilic esophagitis are different than typical reflux symptoms. In reflux symptoms, the feeling is often burning, such as heartburn. However, individuals with eosinophilic esophagitis often have pain after food is swallowed. Over a decade ago, a study was performed in children with a large number of eosinophils in their esophagus, who were not responding well to antireflux medications such as antacids. They were put on a diet that excluded the major allergens and were fed an amino acid–based formula that did not contain whole protein. Within a few weeks, eosinophils in their esophagus had cleared and their symptoms improved. This was the first evidence that large numbers of eosinophils in the esophagus may have represented a disorder different from reflux.

One way that scientists learn about a disease and how to treat it is to use animal models, such as mice, to mimic human disease. One animal model of eosinophilic gastrointestinal disease showed that it was possible to cause an eosinophilic-type inflammation in mice who were made allergic to allergens placed both in the lung and in the stomach. These mice behaved like individuals with allergic eosinophilic gastroenteritis. Experiments on these mice disclosed that particular chemical signals brought the eosinophils into the inflamed areas of the gut. These were important studies because they disclosed that allergens could trigger this type of allergic eosinophilic response. Importantly, particular molecules may be involved that, perhaps if blocked, may reduce the inflammation (aside from trying to remove the allergen that is triggering the problem).

Many studies have shown that by dramatically excluding most foods from the diet, one can reduce the allergic inflammation in the gastrointestinal tract. Unfortunately, these diets tend to be restrictive of large numbers of foods. Physicians and families are essentially working "blindly" because we cannot see what is going on inside of the gastrointestinal tract unless tubes are inserted down the esophagus to perform a biopsy. In addition, it can take weeks for allergic inflammation to fade away if the right diet is achieved, and the allergic inflammation can reappear if the wrong foods are added back to the diet.

Therefore, the diagnosis and treatment of this disorder is particularly difficult and frustrating.

Simple, noninvasive, and accurate diagnostic methods are needed for this disorder. Allergy prick skin tests (described in Chapter 10) are often revealing in trying to diagnose which foods may be problematic, but they are often inconclusive. As described in Chapter 30, allergy patch tests, where food is placed on the skin for days and the area examined for a rash, may help determine which foods may contribute to the problem. However, the diagnostic abilities of these methods are controversial and imperfect. Because of the limitations of these simple tests, trial and error in the dietary management of this disorder is often undertaken.

A child, or an adult, may be placed on a series of very limited diets and evaluated for symptoms. Usually, repeated biopsies are necessary to determine whether the allergic inflammation has cleared during the trial diets. If the allergic inflammation has cleared, one or more foods are typically added to the diet, and time is allowed to pass as symptoms are monitored. Often, a diet can be found that restricts a number of foods but allows a nutritious balance to maintain low, or no, inflammation. Determining a safe diet can be quite arduous and often requires input from a dietitian, allergist, gastroenterologist, and pediatrician. Growth and symptoms are monitored, and biopsies are repeated. The hope is to find a safe, nutritious, balanced, and interesting diet that does not cause inflammation yet supports growth. Some individuals do not respond to diet either because allergy is not a cause or because an airborne allergen, such as pollen, is triggering the illness.

If individuals do not respond well to dietary changes, medicines are prescribed. Steroid medications quiet the immune system responses; eosinophils are sensitive to steroids. If eosinophilic gastrointestinal disease flares, many physicians prescribe oral steroids in liquid or pill form. To reduce possible side effects from steroids—growth problems, sugar imbalance, increased blood pressure, and bone thinning—physicians have tried applying steroids directly to the inflamed area in the intestinal tract, similar to how topical steroids are used on skin rashes or inhaled steroids are used for asthma. Some physicians have had patients use inhaled steroids from canisters like those for asthma, which are sprayed into the mouth and then swallowed. Or they've tried low-dose steroid preparation to treat eosinophilic esophagitis, in which thick gels are swallowed to coat the esophagus. Reports have been mixed on the success of this approach, and side effects have been detected. Some people on this therapy developed fungal infections in the esophagus. Additional anti-allergy medications, including antihistamines and antileukotriene medications, which block specific allergy pathways, have also been tried but their usefulness was unclear.

In animal models of allergic eosinophilic gastrointestinal disease, specific molecules that attract eosinophils to inflamed areas have been identified, and molecules that counter these signaling chemicals have been developed. Preliminary studies indicate that by injecting an individual with these blocking treatments, the eosinophilic inflammation may be reduced.

Eosinophilic gastrointestinal disorders are increasing and represent a difficult allergic illness to diagnose and treat. However, we are learning more about these disorders and improving treatment. Allergic eosinophilic esophagitis may be long-lived given that adults have these disorders as well. Inflammation may result in scarring, or what physicians call "strictures," of the esophagus, which for some adults requires stretching the esophagus to help foods go down. Treating eosinophilic esophagitis, therefore, is in part aimed at reducing inflammation so that these strictures will not develop. Some people question whether the condition could lead to cancer of the esophagus. Fortunately, in studies to date of adults with this disorder, the illness does not appear to be precancerous. Infants who have eosinophilic gut disease have not yet been followed as they mature, to see how often and when the disease resolves.

may be colicky and are more likely to improve if cow's milk is removed from their own diet or the diet of their nursing mother. The literature only partly supports this assumption. Switching a colicky infant to a hypoallergenic infant formula, or *extensive hydrolysate formula* (see Chapter 23), or having a nursing mother avoid milk, may result in improved colic regardless of milk allergy.

Many non-diet-related treatments have been tried for colic. Anti-gas treatments and carrying and holding the infant appear to be ineffective. Reducing stimulation, however, helps 50 percent of infants with colic or reduces symptoms by about half. Some evidence suggests that soy formula or even an herbal tea may be helpful (although tea can cause nutritional deficits in infants). Various studies have evaluated low-allergen diets, in which either a nursing mother avoids typical allergenic foods or a hypoallergenic infant formula replaces breast-feeding. In general, this approach was effective, but only about one-half to one-third as effective as reducing stimulation. These results have led researchers to suggest treatment with reduced stimulation and a weeklong trial on a low-allergen diet. In any event, a link to allergy has not been proved. The good news: colic can disappear spontaneously, even if these dietary measures fail.

Raw Fruits and Vegetables and an Itchy Mouth (Oral Allergy Syndrome / Pollen-Food-Related Syndrome)

Before starting college, 17-year-old Robyn came to my office for an evaluation of multiple food allergies. Her family had noticed that since age 7 she refused raw fruits, such as cherries, peaches, and nectarines. She occasionally ate apples but only certain types, and she would insist that they be peeled. She explained that these foods made her mouth and ears itchy. At the family's urging, she recently tried a peach and developed a more frightening reaction, with lip swelling and severe stomach pain. However, she routinely tolerated canned peaches and applesauce or apple juice with no problem. The family wondered whether these reactions were dangerous and were caused by either the fruit or a fertilizer or chemical sprayed on the fruit.

Robyn was experiencing *oral allergy syndrome*, or *pollen-food-related syndrome*, in which a person first becomes allergic to protein in airborne pollen, such as birch or ragweed pollen, and then experiences allergic reactions to foods that contain similar proteins to those found in the pollen grains. The problem often develops in later childhood or in adulthood after a person has lived through a number of pollen seasons. I was not surprised that hay fever symptoms and mild asthma during the tree pollen season had bothered her for many years and that her tests to birch pollen were positive. The foods she reacted to contain similar proteins to those in birch pollen. Other associations of pollen allergy with fruits and vegetables include:

Pollen	*Food (examples)*
birch	apple, peach, plum, cherry, potato, carrot, hazelnut, pumpkin seed, celery, zucchini
ragweed	melon, banana
mugwort	celery, tomato, honey, chamomile
grass	tomato, melon, peach

Fortunately, reactions to fruits and vegetables are usually mild and limited to the mouth. Itching in the ear canal results from nerve stimulation around the mouth. Typical symptoms also include mild lip swelling. It is uncommon for symptoms to occur beyond the mouth, probably because digestion destroys the pollen-like proteins in these raw foods, and they do not circulate to the rest of the body. That is, the proteins responsible for causing this type of food allergy are easily destroyed by stomach acid and digestion. Similarly, when Robyn ate the cooked forms of the food, such as applesauce, apple juice, or canned peaches, she had no symptoms because heating the foods destroyed the pollen-like proteins. If I performed an allergy skin test on Robyn using fresh juice from a raw apple, it would be positive; however, if I used pasteurized apple juice for the same test, it would be negative because heating during pasteurizing destroyed the problem protein.

Studies performed primarily on adults in Europe show that 7 percent of persons experience some symptoms beyond the mouth, and about 1 percent have severe reactions. Severe reactions seem to occur when the immune system attacks proteins in the same foods which are not pollen-like and are less sensitive to heat, stomach acid, or digestion. In addition, there may be certain circumstances that reduce the body's ability to destroy the protein, leading to more severe reactions. For example, for some people, when foods are eaten with alcohol, before exercise, or in large quantities, a more severe reaction may occur. Apparently, more protein is absorbed unchanged into the bloodstream in these circumstances.

In a study performed by my research group and headed by Dr. Anna Nowak-Wegrzyn, regarding allergist's approach to this syndrome, most took a case-by-case approach to instructions about avoidance. In general, if a person's symptoms were very mild and did not make ingestion unpleasant, and the person wished to eat the foods, restrictions were not imposed. If the foods caused discomfort, the instruction was to avoid them. Not all allergists prescribed emergency medications such as self-injectable epinephrine (1 in 3 never did), but the majority who prescribed it did so on a case-by-case basis. Robyn experienced both mouth and stomach symptoms, generally avoided the foods already, and had asthma, which is a risk factor for more severe reactions. Therefore, I decided that Robyn should have emergency medications available. She tolerated certain types of apples and certain related fruits (pears) and would continue to eat those.

Robyn and her family were advised to watch out for other nuances of this syndrome. Many people assume that fertilizer on the peel of the fruit is the problem, when actually the fruit peel contains more of the causal protein, which is why she tolerated the fruit better when it was peeled. Sometimes the protein in the peel triggers a more severe reaction if it is eaten, another reason I preferred that she not eat the fruit that bothered her. Some people have worse symptoms during or after the pollen season associated with the fruit or vegetable. Robyn was instructed to look for this pattern. Also, some types of apples contain more of the relevant protein than others, which explains Robyn's tolerance of certain apples. Some people describe fewer problems if the fruit is microwaved briefly or soaked in lemon juice; presumably these actions destroy the causal proteins. Finally, most people with this syndrome, for unexplained reasons, tolerate certain related fruits and not others, and so Robyn would not stop ingesting related foods that did not bother her.

Sudden Gastrointestinal Reactions to Foods

Immediate allergic reactions may affect only the gastrointestinal tract, with symptoms such as immediate pain or vomiting and sometimes diarrhea. Unlike FPIES, the reaction begins within minutes and, unlike pollen-food syndrome, with no mouth symptoms. Foods other than raw fruits and vegetables are to blame. These isolated gastrointestinal reactions most often occur in people who experience generalized allergic reactions to a food. In this case, the reaction only affects the gut in a person who on other occasions may experience symptoms in various parts of the body from the same food. Rarely, an individual may experience isolated intestinal symptoms as their only type of reaction to the particular food. The symptoms often mimic intolerance, and typical allergy tests may or may not be positive. In this instance, the allergic response is localized in the stomach and intestines.

Other Gut-Related Food Allergies

Additional gastrointestinal symptoms have been attributed to food allergy, most often to milk. Some studies show that infants and young children with reflux (spitting up, heartburn symptoms) may be milk-responsive. Several studies have linked chronic constipation to an immune response to food. In these cases, constipation improved after certain allergens, usually milk protein, were eliminated. In both of these disorders, causes for the symptoms other than a food-allergic reaction is usually found, and so the role of allergy is somewhat controversial. If food allergy is a cause of constipation, apparently it affects just a subset of persons with these symptoms.

Celiac disease, also called *gluten-sensitive enteropathy,* is caused by an immune system response to gluten, a protein in wheat, and related proteins in barley and rye. This is an inherited disorder where the intestines and other parts of the body may be affected. Nearly 1 in 100 persons has celiac disease. Most experts do not consider celiac disease to be a "food allergy." However, it is an immune system attack associated with a food protein, so it may be considered a type of allergic response. The diagnosis of celiac disease is considered if diarrhea, poor growth, stomach pain, vomiting, constipation, bloating, and irritability are present and also if other family members have been diagnosed with the disease. Sometimes symptoms exist outside of the intestines, for example, poorly developed tooth enamel, blistering skin rashes, and poor bone development. Diagnosis generally requires special blood tests that can be performed by a pediatrician as well as endoscopies and biopsies performed by a pediatric gastroenterologist. Treatment requires a strict gluten-free diet. Unlike most food allergies, celiac disease does not resolve with time and treatment, and it is associated with a risk for cancer.

~

A food allergy can affect the gastrointestinal tract in many ways. Food allergies that affect the intestines of infants without symptoms in other parts of the body are often caused by milk or soy protein and result in three patterns of illness: (1) bloody stools, usually found in a breast-fed infant; (2) poor absorption of nutrients with poor growth and diarrhea; and (3) severe vomiting and diarrhea. These three patterns of illness are not identified by allergy tests that help diagnose sudden food-allergic reactions such as hives or anaphylaxis. Older infants and children may develop allergic inflammation in the gastrointestinal tract, leading to a variety of symptoms and poor intestinal function. These eosinophilic gut disorders often are attributed to multiple food allergies. Colic, spitting up, and constipation may be food related, but whether they are truly "allergies" is unclear. For older children who have become pollen-allergic, it is not uncommon for them to experience an itchy mouth—a pollen-related oral food allergy syndrome—from raw fruits and vegetables that contain proteins similar to the ones in the pollens. Many gastrointestinal problems unrelated to food allergy share symptoms with food-allergic gastrointestinal disorders. Your pediatrician must consider a long list of possibilities if your infant or child is having problems with vomiting and diarrhea. However, some key features, such as increased symptoms with certain foods or resolution of symptoms when the foods are eliminated, and certain patterns of illness I have described, provide clues that indicate a food allergy may be the problem.

5 ~ Breathing Problems

Joshua was only 3 years old, but he had already been hospitalized twice for asthma. Every time he caught a cold, he developed wheezing, a noise made in the lungs when air does not flow out well, and his family felt they had him on too many medications. His pediatrician and pulmonologist had prescribed several inhaled medications. When I saw Joshua, I wondered whether allergy played a part in his asthma. I took a thorough history. Joshua almost always developed a runny nose, red eyes, and coughing when he was around cats. During the tree pollen season, he experienced red eyes, an itchy nose, and wheezing. In winter, especially when he caught a cold, he wheezed and coughed. His medications were maximized, but what could be done about allergic triggers?

Infections, exercise, and irritants such as tobacco smoke are some of the many triggers for asthma. When allergists are considering allergic triggers for asthma, they focus on airborne allergens, such as mold spores, pollens, pet dander, pests such as cockroaches or mice, and dust mites (microscopic insects that live in bedding, stuffed animals, carpeting, and other thick items that can hold some moisture). I asked how these triggers affect Joshua and performed allergy tests that showed positive responses to cat, dust mites, and tree pollen. I advised Joshua's family on how to reduce his exposure to these common allergens, which would likely improve his overall asthma control (see the Glossary of Common Allergic Disorders). But Joshua's family had an additional concern: Could a food allergy be causing his asthma?

A food allergy can be associated with asthma in three ways:

1. A person with a food allergy eats the food and experiences an allergic reaction that may include wheezing.

2. The food to which there is an allergy is inhaled directly.

3. A person is routinely eating a food to which they are allergic and this causes frequent and continuous symptoms of asthma.

There have been studies and reports about each of these possible problems.

Episodes of Asthma in Children with Food Allergies

A child with an allergic disposition might experience allergic problems such as allergic skin rashes (atopic dermatitis, eczema), hay fever, asthma, and allergies to foods and airborne allergens. Studies have shown that among asthmatic children, about 1 in 10–20 experience food allergy, in which ingestion of the problematic food results in wheezing, usually in combination with other symptoms, such as hives. If children have a more intense allergy history, say, asthma and a history of wheezing associated with a particular food or foods, then evaluations typically confirm a food-induced asthma response in 1 in 3–4 such children. During an allergic reaction to a food, nearly 1 in 5 children experience symptoms of lung obstruction, such as coughing and wheezing and increased rate of breathing.

According to Joshua's parents, he'd never had an allergic reaction to any food he had eaten. In fact, he had been eating many allergenic foods, such as milk, egg, seafood, and peanut, without a problem. Given that even among children with food allergies, food-related wheezing reactions are relatively uncommon, I did not suspect Joshua had food allergy.

Inhalation Reactions

Suppose a child is allergic to a food, has asthma, and inhales airborne food particles from the food to which he is allergic. Medical literature on this subject reveals that common reactions from air exposure typically occur while food is being cooked because cooking releases food-protein particles into the air (e.g., cooking bean soup, scrambling eggs, boiling milk, and frying fish). In these situations, one can usually see the steam rising from the foods. Respiratory reactions are typical, such as hay fever symptoms of red, itchy eyes, runny nose, and then coughing and wheezing. These symptoms are usually no different from reactions to other airborne allergens. For example, Joshua had experienced these same symptoms around cats and during the pollen season. In some circumstances, food allergens become airborne without heating. This includes dust from loose dry-roasted peanuts, fish proteins in a fish market, and powdery versions of foods such as dry milk and flour (wheat, soy, peanut, etc.). Asthma may be associated with occupational exposures to foods (such a reaction to wheat is called *baker's asthma).* In contrast to these special circumstances, food proteins usually do not emanate from finished foods, oily foods, or cooled foods, for example, a cooled serving of fish, a glass of milk, peanut butter, and so on.

In a study my research team conducted, none of thirty children with severe peanut allergy reacted to sniffing peanut butter for ten minutes. Another group of researchers undertook a study to determine how children respond to airborne food particles during cooking. The researchers were able to induce a reaction in 9 of 12 children who had both asthma and a prior history of a reaction when near a food to which they were allergic while it was being cooked. During the study, children developed asthma symptoms when they were close to the following foods as they were cooked: fish, chickpea, milk, egg, and buckwheat. One child who reacted to buckwheat had hives as well as asthma. These results indicate that airborne food particles, like other airborne allergens, can cause asthmatic reactions when the amount in the air is high (close proximity to cooking). These reactions are similar to ones that occur when persons with other airborne allergies, such as cat allergy, inhale large amounts of these proteins. An episode of asthma can occur; however, anaphylaxis would be a very unusual response.

Food Allergy and Chronic Asthma

Joshua's family was concerned that he might be eating an "asthma-causing" food. They had focused on cow's milk because of the belief that milk caused mucus and with asthma, extra mucus is present in the lung. I explained to Joshua's parents that in studies in which the ingestion of a food was linked to asthma, the child usually had additional food allergy symptoms, such as vomiting, diarrhea, poor growth, and skin problems, such as atopic dermatitis. It was unlikely that foods would be an issue for Joshua's asthma because he never had a reaction to a food and had no other symptoms of food allergy; however, he did have clear-cut symptoms associated with pollen, dust mite, and cat dander exposure. I encouraged Joshua's family to limit his exposure to these allergens and to continue his asthma medications.

The situation was different for Maria, a 5-year-old with asthma and atopic dermatitis who had known severe reactions to peanuts, tree nuts, and shellfish. She came to my office primarily because her asthma and skin rashes were severe and required daily medications. Her condition was worsening despite these medications and appropriate environmental changes to reduce exposures to airborne allergens. Maria had already been tested for allergies, which confirmed peanut, tree nut, and seafood allergies and allergies to dust, cat, dog, and pollens. A careful review of her diet revealed that she did not like to eat most milk or egg products and that she had reacted to these foods during the previous year. Her diet history showed that, although she did not eat eggs or drink milk, she did have food in her diet that contained modest amounts of these common allergenic food proteins. For example, she ate small amounts of foods containing egg (pasta, French toast, mayonnaise) and milk (cheeses and some ice cream).

I explained to Maria's family that nearly half of the children with problems like Maria's develop "twitchy" airways when they eat the food to which they are allergic. Maria was not avoiding milk or egg but ate a small amount, possibly not enough to trigger more obvious allergic reactions. Maria's allergy tests were positive for milk and egg. During a feeding test, I fed her larger amounts of these two foods than she usually consumed, and she developed obvious allergic symptoms, including coughing and increased atopic dermatitis. After these foods were eliminated from her diet, her skin rashes and asthma improved significantly. She still needed medications and had to avoid the airborne allergens that troubled her, but she needed less medication and had fewer symptoms.

Nasal Problems

Irwin was a 15-month-old brought to my office by his father to be evaluated for a possible milk allergy that caused a runny nose. According to his father, Irwin had not experienced any typical allergic problems except when he drank milk. The family noticed he would develop a clear nasal drip when he ingested milk.

I explained to the family that research studies show that having isolated nasal symptoms from a food allergy is extremely unlikely. During food-allergic reactions, it is common to experience hay fever–type symptoms such as nasal congestion, itch, a clear drip, and sneezing. However, with food-allergic reactions, these nasal symptoms do not generally occur without additional symptoms in other parts of the body; for example, there may be simultaneous rashes and gastrointestinal symptoms. Many conditions can cause a congested and runny nose, including the common cold or a virus. A doctor must consider numerous reasons for nasal symptoms, including infections and bone abnormalities. However, itch and sneeze, drip and congestion, are typical allergy symptoms. These allergic nasal symptoms are usually triggered by pollen, animal dander, and other environmental allergens. Food does not usually cause chronic nasal symptoms.

Irwin's nose was usually just fine; it only became trouble when he drank milk. Because there were no chronic or seasonal symptoms, I did not consider testing for environmental allergens such as dust mite, cat, or pollen. I performed an allergy test that was slightly positive to milk. I had Irwin take a drink of milk under my supervision. Irwin's head rested on his dad's shoulder. I noticed a circle of wetness on his father's shirt. Irwin was that rare baby who seemed to have only nasal symptoms from milk allergy. I saw him a year later, and fortunately he tolerated milk with no symptoms at all.

Other Breathing Problems

Although many grandmothers explain that milk causes "mucus," there are inadequate studies to prove whether grandmothers are correct. I usually suggest a short trial of reducing milk consumption if there are concerns about this issue. During viral respiratory infections that cause a lot of nasal congestion and mucus, young children often prefer thin fluids such as juices and tea, rather than milk or milk products.

Heiner's syndrome is a rare type of allergy to milk. Babies with this disorder develop bleeding in the lungs and lung failure related to an immune reaction to milk protein. The reaction is not like typical allergy (no hives, etc.), and typical allergy tests are negative.

~

It is not common to have daily asthma or daily nasal problems from foods. However, during a sudden allergic reaction to food, the nose and lungs are often briefly affected as part of a generalized allergic reaction. For a person who has asthma and a food allergy, inhalation of food particles can result in hay fever and asthma symptoms similar to how other airborne allergens, such as pollen and animal dander, may cause these symptoms in children allergic to those allergens. For foods to become a relevant airborne allergen, proteins need to be released into the air, for example, during cooking.

6 ~ Growth Problems

Children grow quickly, gaining height and weight in leaps and bounds that your pediatrician records on "growth curves." A child may not gain weight or grow as expected for many reasons. Food allergy is one of many possibilities. It is probably no surprise that food allergy affecting the intestines could result in poor growth, but it is also possible for food allergy to cause poor growth even if there are no gastrointestinal symptoms. In this chapter, we consider some ways that food allergy could affect growth.

Danny was 18 months old when it became distressingly clear that he was not growing well. His pediatrician had been charting his height and weight on a growth chart and noted that at 9 months, his weight gain had been decreasing. Nearly nine months later, despite a calorie-rich diet, he had continued to do poorly and had no weight gain for almost two months. His height had remained normal for his age, but he was quite thin. His pediatrician sent Danny to me because he had significant atopic dermatitis. Danny was also evaluated by a gastroenterologist who was treating him for reflux with a medication that appeared to be working well because his frequent episodes of spitting up had declined.

I carefully evaluated Danny's diet history. Danny had never experienced a sudden or severe food-allergic reaction, but his family noticed that egg and milk made his rash worse, so they limited the amount of these foods in his diet. They had not fed Danny peanut or fish because several family members were allergic to these foods. He was also a picky eater, and mealtimes sometimes lasted for hours. His skin rashes were fairly severe, and more than half of his body was red, itchy, and peeling. A dermatologist had advised using topical steroids, but Danny's family was reluctant because they feared steroids could further suppress his growth. I noted that the decline in his weight and his reflux symptoms developed *after* he discontinued breast-feeding and added a variety of foods as well as a milk- and then soy-based formula to his diet.

When evaluating an infant or child with poor growth, the pediatrician must consider a number of possibilities. The pediatrician may first evaluate whether weight, height, or both are affected and then consider everything from mild problems such as poor caloric intake or normal growth delays to more serious conditions including genetic diseases, heart or blood problems, organ failure, digestion problems, infections, immune system disorders, and cancer. Among these conditions, food allergy may deserve consideration, though it is not the most common reason for poor weight gain.

In Danny's case, the clues that led his pediatrician and me to suspect food allergy as a cause for his poor weight gain were his atopic dermatitis and reflux; both are possible food-allergy-related disorders. In addition, his family had noticed his rash worsened with certain foods. And because allergies are inherited, the family history of allergies meant that his risk for having allergies increased as well. Danny's growth problems began when his diet was broadened to include an increased number of allergenic foods, another reason to suspect food allergy.

To ensure we appropriately solved Danny's troubles, we considered two issues. First, it was important that alternative explanations for his problems were ruled out. Second, we needed to identify which foods might be problematic.

Danny's pediatrician had already performed some blood screening tests to exclude possible medical causes for his poor weight gain. My concern was that the culprit could be several illnesses characterized by skin rashes and poor growth but that have nothing to do with food allergies, and we would not want to miss those problems. He did not have evidence of these diseases, however, according to tests done by his pediatrician, dermatologist, and gastroenterologist. Sometimes a gastroenterologist will do specialized tests, for example, an endoscopy. In an endoscopy, a tube with a camera and a "pincer" that can grab a bit of the lining of the gastrointestinal tract (to examine under a microscope) is placed through the mouth or nose into the upper intestine or up through the anus to evaluate the lower intestine. However, we decided not to perform this procedure on Danny.

I focused on food allergy. Several studies have shown that children with food-responsive atopic dermatitis often have problems with absorption of nutrients from the intestine, as though a rash inside of the digestive tract hinders a child's ability to absorb calories. Danny had evidence of a gastrointestinal problem because he had been vomiting. In addition, Danny had problems with weight gain, not growth in height. Many illnesses affect height and weight or even height alone; however, when the body has trouble absorbing calories, weight loss is typical while height is preserved. In addition to the high likelihood that Danny's gastrointestinal tract was not working efficiently if he was ingesting foods to which he was allergic, it was also likely that his skin condition was using up a lot of his calories. When a child has severe atopic dermatitis, the skin has to repair itself continuously, which expends a lot of energy. Improved skin care would likely save calories for Danny.

Danny's parents were concerned about his picky eating. Picky eating is normal for toddlers, who often like to eat the same foods over and over. But this symptom should not be ignored when other signs of food allergy exist. So, picky eating may be normal, but if weight loss is an issue, it becomes more significant. When I see a child with atopic dermatitis, reflux, and "pickiness," it suggests that eating has become a discomfort or that particular foods have caused reactions that prevent the child from enjoying a varied diet. Perhaps Danny had learned to avoid certain foods. About 50 percent of young children who refuse to eat peanut and are found to have a positive allergy test to peanut react if they are *forced* to eat it. Sometimes a child loses interest in eating because of chronic discomfort caused by swelling and inflammation in their gastrointestinal tract triggered by a food they eat frequently. Another way food refusal may develop is if a child is scared by a dramatic adverse reaction to a food, leading the child to fear eating foods or trying new foods. I discovered that Danny did not really refuse foods in general, only certain foods, and we learned that the ones he didn't like usually contained larger amounts of milk or egg.

I had a dietitian carefully evaluate Danny's daily diet. This revealed that Danny was ingesting an appropriate number of calories for his age and size. Because caloric intake was appropriate, the possibility that his poor weight gain was from poor intake was excluded. I was correct that poor calorie absorption and increased needs from his skin rash were the major issues accounting for his growth problems. Allergy tests identified several foods in his diet that were likely problematic, including egg and milk. With limits to his diet and increased use of skin medications, he gained weight. Even though he was eating a smaller variety of foods, his appetite improved, possibly because the foods that remained in his diet were not bothering him. His reflux symptoms were gone and did not recur during a trial respite from reflux medications, and his skin was easier to manage with fewer treatments. Within a month, Danny gained significant weight and was feeling better.

Danny's family reported that his behavior improved, and he was happier and less irritable.

Poor growth in weight and sometimes height can be caused by food allergy. Your pediatrician will consider many other possible causes as well because food allergy is not a common reason for failure of an infant or young child to grow properly. Additional evaluation by a gastroenterologist and dietitian is often needed.

7 ~ Behavior and Developmental Disabilities

The most common manifestations of food allergy are allergic skin rashes, intestinal diseases, and sudden allergic reactions with symptoms such as hives or breathing problems. However, other problems—from headaches to temper tantrums, seizures to arthritis—have been attributed to food allergy. Many of these illnesses or problems have not been clearly linked to a food allergy. In some cases, nonallergic reactions to foods may be a factor. For example, a few reports show persons with seizures or epilepsy seemed to have fewer seizures on special diets. No evidence suggests that seizures are a result of a food allergy; however, special diets, called *ketogenic* diets, reduce the number of seizures for certain types of epilepsy. In older persons with arthritis, some reports suggest dietary changes can relieve the arthritis. Again, these rare associations probably do not result from allergy but are, perhaps, a response to changes in other pharmacologic or chemical dietary aspects or may be random associations.

In children, food "allergy" is blamed for a number of behavior or developmental problems, but this notion is a bit controversial. One clear way that food allergy can affect behavior is through the medical illness, such as skin or intestinal problems, caused by the allergy. For example, many parents notice that their children "behaved" when they avoided allergenic foods that caused rashes. If you have a headache or stomachache or have an illness that disrupts sleep, the discomfort will naturally affect you. You may have trouble enjoying an activity, feel irritable or unhappy, or be more likely to lash out at someone. In regard to allergic disease, chronic nasal symptoms, skin itchiness, stomach problems, or asthma can interfere with enjoying normal daily activities, and treating these problems is known to improve quality of life and behavior.

In contrast to these expected relationships of behavior to food-allergic diseases, many behavioral problems and developmental disorders have been variably attributed to reactions to foods where the relationship to a food allergy is not clear. In this chapter, we explore the role of adverse reactions to foods in hyperactivity and autism.

Hyperactivity

JoAnne saw me for an allergy evaluation because her parents suspected a wheat allergy. A 7-year-old who had trouble with attention and concentration in school and other situations, JoAnne seemed to move quickly from activity to activity without being able to focus on the task at hand. Her pediatrician suggested medications for attention deficit–hyperactivity disorder, and this medication was effective. However, JoAnne's parents suspected that she had a wheat allergy because after consuming certain dietary products with wheat, she became more "active" and aggressive and even less attentive than usual.

I explained to JoAnne's parents that there have been a variety of theories regarding the role of diet in hyperactivity and attention problems. Very commonly, "sugar" has been implicated. The classic story is that a child eats a food with high sugar content and then becomes more active or aggressive. However, in carefully conducted studies of children whose families suspected this problem, no adverse changes in behavior could be documented when the children were on high-, low-, or no-added sugar diets. To conduct these studies, the sugar content of foods was hidden. Diets were randomly provided without the family, child, or observers knowing which diet was used at a particular time under evaluation.

The medical and lay literature includes both personal stories and research studies regarding possible adverse effects of food dyes and preservatives on behavior. These additives and preservatives are generally not thought to stimulate an adverse immune response (food allergy), but most of the concern regards a possible pharmacologic (chemical) effect on behavior. The jury is still out on whether food additives affect behavior. In studies where families or children were aware that food additives were in their foods, problems were noted to a greater extent than when this fact was hidden from them. This indicates that subjective expectations play a role in behavior. Some well-designed studies appear to show adverse effects of food additives on behavior contributing to hyperactivy. Although final conclusions may be lacking, at least a subset of children may be affected. However, certain food components have clear pharmacologic effects (e.g., caffeine, which is found in many candies and sodas).

In JoAnne's situation, I explained that in the absence of any typical allergic symptoms, and no wheat allergy symptoms in particular, wheat was probably not the problem. The family still wanted to evaluate this possibility, so with the help of my dietitian, a test was implemented. Muffins with and without wheat were prepared. JoAnne would receive one batch of muffins during one week and another during the next week. Her family and teachers would monitor the reactions. Neither her family nor I would know in which week she was receiving the wheat muffins.

After one muffin, her family called me to say that a wheat reaction had occurred. After the muffin, she began hitting her brother and was quite uncontrollable. I suggested they not give her more muffins and wait for the new batch of muffins the following week. After one muffin from the next batch, the same problem occurred. Because wheat was in only one of the muffins, the wheat was not the cause of JoAnne's behavior.

Autism

Seven-year-old Michael was diagnosed with autism (pervasive developmental disorder). His family requested an evaluation with tests for food allergy to see whether allergy was a factor in his developmental problems.

Autism is a chronic condition characterized by variable problems with sociability and verbal and nonverbal communication, as well as a reduced range of interests and activities. Children with autism may have behavioral disturbances, stereotyped behavior, and mental retardation. The specific features can vary widely in type and severity. Only a few studies of the possible adverse role of foods in autism have been conducted.

Allergy is often used to describe the association of developmental problems with foods, in particular, with milk (casein) and wheat. In published studies to date, only small groups of children have been evaluated, and the studies were limited because either the diets were not "disguised" from people observing the children, there was no comparison group of children who were not on the diets, or both. Overall, improvement attributable to the diet was unconvincing. Some children with autism reportedly have gastrointestinal inflammation, which has led researchers to consider a relationship between intestinal inflammation and autism, including the possible role of food allergy. However, the gastrointestinal problems described were not similar to ones seen in typical allergy, and subsequent studies indicated that about the same proportion of children without autism as with autism had this type of bowel problem. Some families believe that excluding particular foods helps their child, and no studies have proved otherwise. The theory relating food and behavior or development in autism generally concerns a pharmacologic influence of the foods rather than an immune response (allergy).

I cautioned Michael's family that a food reaction as a cause or contributor to autism had not been proved. About the same proportion of children with autism have typical allergies and food allergies as children without autism. For children with autism who have typical food allergies, safe diets must be implemented. However, the relationship between diet changes and behavior and development is less clear. Altering the diet can be risky for anyone because of nutritional deficits and social issues. Children with autism often have fixed food preferences, and Michael indeed displayed these preferences, so altering his diet would not be easy and could carry a risk of more behavioral problems. Performing typical allergy tests to evaluate possible food triggers in autism was not a reasonable option. Instead, only eliminating and readministering foods could be offered. But which foods should be eliminated? I discussed with Michael's family that prior studies primarily addressed the elimination of milk and wheat.

I worry that families may place an inordinate value on diet changes for treatment in autism. To give one example, the parents of a child with autism removed milk from the child's diet. Several months later, the child said a new word. This led the family to remove additional foods from the diet at the risk of nutritional deficits.

I supported the wish of Michael's family to undertake a diet trial, but I explained the limitations of current studies and warned them about potential placebo effects and nutritional risks of diet changes. I advised them not to notify Michael's teachers about diet changes and to see whether they remarked on any strong improvements. Also, the family would need to decide on the level of improvement they were going to look for and what would make them decide that a diet was helpful. Ultimately, Michael did not appear to benefit from a casein and wheat-free diet.

Food allergy can lead to chronic disease that can affect behavior. However, food allergy is often perceived as a factor in many behavioral and developmental disorders where it is not likely to be an issue. In disorders such as hyperactivity, behavioral problems, attention deficit, and autism, nonimmunological adverse reactions to pharmacologically active elements in foods has been considered a potential cause or contributor to these disorders. Unfortunately, definitive studies are lacking, and the area remains controversial. In many situations, trial diets are needed to determine potential relationships, but these are difficult to interpret because symptoms are often subjective and can easily be a placebo effect. If such diet trials are undertaken, they should be done under supervision so that nutritional needs are fulfilled and an additional opinion on outcomes can be obtained.

8 ~ Additives and Cross-Reactions

When your child has been diagnosed with an allergy to a particular food, it is natural for you to wonder whether other foods may become a problem. The concern usually arises because your child has not yet eaten a particular food or because your child has an allergy to a food and you are worried about "related" foods.

Eggs, milk, peanuts, wheat, soy, tree nuts (e.g., walnuts, pecans), and seafood (fish and shellfish) account for nearly 90 percent of the problems. These foods and food groups, sometimes along with seeds, are termed the *major food allergens.* Although food protein is the target for an immune system "attack" that can lead to allergies, it is not just a food high in protein such as egg or fish that can cause an allergic reaction. All foods have protein, and almost every food has been reported to cause a reaction for someone. It is believed that the reason just a few foods cause so much trouble is that the proteins in these "major allergens" are more likely to survive digestion and to trigger an immune reaction. Not only are some foods more likely to be responsible for allergies, but certain foods—like peanuts, tree nuts, and seafood—are more likely than others to cause severe allergic reactions. It follows, then, that a child who is allergic to milk is unlikely to be allergic to, say, squash. However, a child who is allergic to milk may be allergic to peanuts, and that possibility is something to be concerned about.

Many related foods share similar proteins. The risk of a child having true allergies to the related ones is variable and depends on the specific type of food. In this chapter, we explore features of the major food allergens, other foods that can cause allergic reactions, and issues regarding cross-reactivity of foods.

I will also address adverse reactions to food additives. An unexplained allergic reaction may be attributed to a chemical additive in the food. Occasionally, the immune system may recognize or be affected by these components of our foods. Many chemical additives are used to preserve, to enhance flavor or texture, or to color our foods. These agents are capable of causing adverse reactions, though not always allergic reactions.

Common Allergenic Foods

Peanuts

Although "nut" is part of "peanut," peanuts are actually related to beans, such as peas and soy. Studies conducted by my colleagues and me and the Food Allergy & Anaphylaxis Network indicate that 1.5 million Americans have a peanut allergy. Peanuts are notorious as an allergen that can trigger severe reactions, although mild allergy is also described. Ninety-five percent of children with a peanut allergy tolerate other legumes (beans), such as peas and string beans.

In Mediterranean countries, allergies to specific beans, namely, lentil and chickpea (garbanzo), are common, but these beans do not commonly present a problem in the United States. In France and several other European countries, lupine or lupin, is eaten as a bean or used to make flour for breads or pasta. Roughly half of peanut-allergic persons in those countries have reacted to lupine, though it has not been a prominent problem in the United States, where lupine is not as widely consumed. However, lupine's popularity is growing, and it may become more prominent as an allergen.

If a person with a peanut allergy is allergy "tested" to other beans, these tests are positive nearly half of the time, but actual reactions to the other beans occur only 5 percent of the time. About 20 percent of young children outgrow a peanut allergy by school age. Highly processed peanut oil contains virtually no protein; it is essentially fat and is not expected to induce a reaction. However, cold-pressed peanut oil contains peanut protein and would pose a danger for a person with peanut allergy. It is usually not easy to know what type of peanut oil is used in various products, so I generally advise patients to avoid peanut oil. If a child with peanut allergy accidentally consumes peanut oil without a reaction, I would not trust that as a sign that perhaps the allergy was gone because there was not likely to be any, or enough, peanut protein in the oil to reach that conclusion.

Tree Nuts

Tree nuts grow on trees and are not related to peanuts. Examples of tree nuts are walnuts, Brazil nuts, hazelnuts, pistachios, pecans, pine nuts, cashews, and macadamia nuts. An allergy to one tree nut does not necessarily mean an allergy to others, though often this is the case. In particular, cashew and pistachio allergy usually coexist, as do walnut and pecan. Almond is usually "counted" as a tree nut, although it is related to apples and pitted fruits. Coconut is often not thought of as a tree nut, but it shares some proteins with walnut. Even so, coconut allergy is not common. Nutmeg and water chestnuts are not nuts. When I have diagnosed a tree nut allergy, I often instruct that all nuts should be avoided because they may be cross-contacted or mixed in many foods from bakeries, ice cream shops, and restaurants. However, if a particular nut is tolerated, it should be safe to eat if it is certain that the problematic nut or nuts to which your child is allergic are not mixed in. An allergy to a tree nut is often persistent, with studies showing that only about 1–2 in 20 children outgrow the allergy during early childhood. Nut oils generally contain the nut protein.

Seeds

Sesame and poppy seeds have been implicated in severe allergic reactions. Other seeds include sunflower, rapeseed, and flaxseed. The oils of these seeds may contain variable amounts of proteins. Like any foods, the quantity ingested is relevant to whether an allergic reaction develops. For example, some people tolerate a few sesame seeds on a slice of bread but have a reaction if they eat tahini, which is solid sesame seed paste and has much larger amounts of protein.

Egg

Chicken egg allergy is estimated to affect about 1 in 50 children, but most tolerate the food by age 5 years. It is presumed that other bird eggs would also cause reactions for those allergic to hen's egg, but this has not been extensively studied. The white part of the egg is the major allergenic portion. Sometimes doctors test for allergy to egg yolk and egg white separately, but testing for the egg yolk is impractical because the egg white is usually in most egg products and the white and yellow are not easily separated.

Cow's Milk

Milk allergy is estimated to affect about 1 in 50 children. If a child is allergic to cow's milk, it is highly likely that the child will be allergic to other mammal milk, such as goat's or sheep's milk. Mare's milk is less likely to cause a reaction but is not a common commercial milk. It is also possible to be allergic to just one type of mammalian milk, for example, to goat's or sheep's milk without being allergic to cow's milk. Sometimes a child will have an allergic reaction to a cheese derived from these mammal milks, even though they have tolerated cow's milk and cow's milk products. Beef retains some cow's milk proteins, and roughly 10 percent of children with a severe cow's milk allergy will have an allergic reaction to beef, particularly if it is not cooked well. Milk allergy is typically outgrown by age 5 years.

Soy

Soy is a legume like peanut and peas. Soy allergy occurs in about 1 in 200 children but is usually outgrown. Like peanut allergy, most persons with a soy allergy do not have allergies to other beans. Soy oil generally has extremely low amounts of residual soy protein and in several studies, typically has been tolerated by persons with soy allergy. Similarly, soy lecithin, a fatty derivative of soy, has trace soy protein and is usually tolerated by persons with soy allergy. Soy sauce, a soy product that has undergone a tremendous amount of fermentation, often has very low amounts of allergenic soy protein, but the amount can vary. Because the amount of soy protein in soy sauce is typically low, if a child has tolerated soy sauce, I do not consider this proof that soy protein would be tolerated.

Wheat

About 1 in 250 children has a wheat allergy. Having a wheat allergy does not necessarily mean there will be another grain allergy, though about 20 percent of children with a wheat allergy have other grain allergies (barley, rye). Most children outgrow their wheat allergy by age 5. *Spelt* is an ancient form of wheat, but the immune system usually reacts to it the same as wheat. *Celiac disease* is distinct from typical food allergies and is associated with gluten in various grains such as wheat, barley, and rye. Oat and rice are not immunologically strongly related to wheat. Buckwheat has been associated with severe reactions, primarily in Japan where it is used widely.

Fish

Finned fish include tuna, salmon, codfish, and many others. Roughly 50 percent of persons allergic to one type of finned fish have multiple fish allergies. Because fish allergy is often severe, many allergists advise avoiding all finned fish. However, some individuals tolerate certain fish, and some persons have an allergy to a single type of fish and no others. Canned forms of tuna or salmon seem less likely to be allergenic than fresh-cooked fish, and canned tuna or salmon is often, but not always, tolerated by persons with a fish allergy. Two percent to 5 percent of young children outgrow a fish allergy.

Shellfish

Crustacean shellfish such as lobster, shrimp, and crab are notorious for causing severe reactions. About 75 percent of persons will react to more than one type of shellfish. Molluscan shellfish (squid) and bivalves (clam, mussel) are less commonly problematic compared with the crustaceans but may also cause reactions. Only about 2 percent to 5 percent of children may outgrow these allergies. Shellfish allergens are similar to allergens in dust mites and cockroaches, presumably because they share ancient ancestry. But it is not clear whether dust mite allergy increases the risk of shellfish allergy. Nonetheless, it is possible for a person with dust mite allergy to test positive for shellfish allergy even though she can tolerate shellfish.

Less Common Allergenic Foods

Fruits and Vegetables

The most common fruit or vegetable allergy is *oral allergy syndrome,* or *pollen-food-related syndrome* (discussed in Chapter 4), which occurs because these foods share proteins with certain pollens a child may have developed an allergy to. While this type of allergy is usually mild and consists primarily of an itchy mouth, it is also possible to have the immune system attack non-pollen-related proteins in fruits and vegetables, which may result in more severe reactions. Even though many fruits and vegetables share similar proteins (e.g., apple, pear, and peach), some children react to just one type, while others may have reactions from several related fruits and vegetables. See page 298 on latex-related food allergies.

Meats

Like fruit and vegetable allergy, reactions to meats, such as poultry (turkey and chicken) and mammalian meats (beef, pork, lamb), is relatively uncommon, and reaction to one meat does not *necessarily* indicate a reaction to related ones. Nonetheless, if a person is allergic to chicken, there is a higher risk than usual of reaction to other poultry, which also holds true for mammalian meats (beef, pork, lamb).

Spices

Spice is often used to describe a variety of flavoring agents, most of which are not spicy or hot (e.g., allspice [a type of pepper], basil, cardamom, celery, chives, cinnamon, coriander, cumin, dill, fennel, garlic, ginger, marjoram, nutmeg, onion, oregano, parsley, pepper, peppermint, rosemary, saffron, sage, savory, star anise, tarragon, turmeric, and vanilla). Many seeds (poppy, sesame, caraway, and mustard) are considered spices. Many types of pepper are used for spice (e.g., bell, red, and cayenne). All of these spices represent an array of food types whose proteins share features with various foods and pollens. Therefore, this large group could be expected to include allergens. Indeed, virtually every spice has been a culprit for causing an allergic reaction, but even when considered as a group, it is estimated that fewer than 1 in 50 persons has a spice allergy. Variations in how a spice is processed (roasted, heated, raw) and the amount in a given food may affect whether the spice will cause a problem for a given individual. "Hot" spices can be tricky because they contain capsaicin, a chemical that triggers a burning sensation in normal individuals that could be misinterpreted as an allergic reaction, especially in children.

Food Additives

A variety of substances are added to foods for flavor, preservation, color, or texture. In the United States, these additives may be listed in order of predominance in a product and sometimes are listed under a collective name such as "spices" or "natural flavor." When a substance is used to process a food but is not part of the final product, the substance might not be listed as an ingredient. For example, boiler water additives used to create steam for food processing need not be labeled as an ingredient. Several studies have investigated the prevalence of allergic reactions to food additives, and typical results indicate fewer than 1 in 500 persons is affected. These substances may likely not cause problems because many are not proteins and are often used in small quantities.

Certain food additives are derived from natural sources and therefore contain proteins. These additives may be more likely to cause typical allergic reactions. Chemical additives are not likely to cause typical allergic reactions, but some may have drug effects that cause adverse reactions, including allergy-like symptoms.

The following discussion is not exhaustive but summarizes features of several food additives that are more commonly used and attributed to adverse food reactions.

Synthetic Colors

Tartrazine (Yellow No. 5) is a synthetic color that has been extensively investigated because of concerns that it may trigger hives, allergic reactions, and asthma. However, well-conducted studies have not validated these concerns. There have been reports of persons who have developed a nonallergic rash from this colorant, including a child whose atopic dermatitis apparently flared when the child ingested large amounts of Yellow No. 5.

Like tartrazine, many other synthetic colors (sunset yellow, erythrosine, ponceau 4R, carmoisine, quinoline yellow, patent blue, and others) have not been proved to cause allergic reactions. Some of these chemicals have been associated with illnesses on rare occasions (rashes, blood vessel disorders) but not typical allergic symptoms.

Natural Colors

Natural colors derive from foods such as turmeric, paprika, beet, and grape skin extract. Annatto is a color obtained from the seed of *Bixa orellana,* a South American tree. The extract gives food an orange or yellow color. Annatto has rarely been associated with typical and anaphylactic allergic reactions. Carmine (cochineal) colors food red. This natural color is derived from dried bodies of a female insect that lives as a parasite on cactus. Aside from the rather unusual and admittedly distasteful origin of this color, it has also rarely been associated with typical allergic reactions.

Chemical Additives

Sulfites

Sulfites are added to foods as a preservative, an antibrowning agent, or to provide a bleaching effect. Before 1986, sulfites were used more widely and in larger amounts, particularly on fresh foods such as lettuce. Sulfites can, in sensitive persons, induce asthma. The asthma response is not believed to be a typical allergic response but rather a chemical effect. The more sulfite in a food, the more likely asthma could result. With regard to more typical allergic reactions, such as hives or anaphylaxis, well-designed studies usually do not confirm such reactions even when they have been suspected by participants. However, a few reports show individuals who appear to have typical allergic reactions to sulfites. Higher amounts of sulfites may be found in dried fruit, lemon juice, sauerkraut, wine vinegar, certain gravies, dried potato, and maraschino cherries, among other foods. Sulfites are listed on package labels.

Sulfites are used to preserve some drugs and occasionally have been associated with triggering asthma. Epinephrine used to treat anaphylaxis has sulfites, but in low amounts that have never been reported to cause a problem (so epinephrine should never be withheld from a person sensitive to sulfites).

Monosodium Glutamate (MSG)

This flavor enhancer occurs naturally in many foods or can be used as an additive. The symptoms attributed to this additive include burning sensations, tingling, headaches, and drowsiness. Numerous well-designed studies have not been able to uniformly reproduce these symptoms in persons believed to be affected. The response is not thought to be allergic in nature.

Benzoates and Parabens

These preservatives have been implicated in various allergic-type reactions, including anaphylaxis. Though very rare, these reactions may represent a true allergic reaction.

Other Chemical Additives

Several other additives appear to cause allergic-type reactions, but carefully conducted studies usually do not implicate them: BHA/BHT (preservatives), nitrites and nitrates (curing agents), sorbates/sorbic acid (preservative), and aspartame (sweetener). Allergic-type reactions to most food additives are rare and, if suspected, should be carefully evaluated. Usually, the suspicion is not confirmed and diet restrictions can, therefore, be avoided.

Natural Additives

When additives derive from foods, proteins are often present that can induce typical allergy responses. Papain, an enzyme used as a meat tenderizer, has rarely induced an allergic reaction. Various gums, such as carrageenan, xanthan, guar, acacia, and locust bean, are derived often from beans and may contain some proteins. Lactose is a milk sugar, but there may be occasions where contamination with milk proteins can occur.

Gelatin is derived mostly from beef or pork and sometimes from fish. It can be a tricky potential allergen because gelatin may be modified during processing, which could affect how it behaves as an allergen. In addition, the amount of gelatin can vary. For example, I have had patients who tolerate gelatin desserts but react to gelatin in candy chews or yogurts. Reactions to gelatin-containing foods is generally uncommon. A child could have allergic reactions to gelatin in childhood vaccines (such as the measles-mumps-rubella vaccine), but the amount of gelatin and its allergenicity may vary by type of vaccine and manufacturer. Usually, a person with beef or pork gelatin allergy can tolerate fish gelatin (found, for example, in kosher gelatin). However, residual fish proteins in fish gelatin may be a problem for those with fish allergy.

Most significant allergic reactions to foods are attributable to milk, egg, peanuts, tree nuts, fish, shellfish, wheat, and soy. These foods, perhaps with the addition of seeds such as sesame, are the major food allergens. However, any food can cause an allergic reaction in some persons. Allergy to one food may increase the chance of a reaction to another food with similar proteins, but the degree of cross-reaction varies by the exact type of food. Allergy to chemical additives is rare, though some are associated with nonallergic adverse reactions. Natural food additives and most spices contain proteins that can occasionally induce an allergic reaction.

PART 2

DIAGNOSING A FOOD ALLERGY

Perhaps your child has experienced an allergic reaction during a meal and you are not certain of the cause. Maybe your child has a chronic health condition such as severe rashes and you would like to know whether foods are responsible. Or you may know that your child has a food allergy and wonder whether the allergy is severe or has been outgrown. For answers, you would ask your doctor to perform a test to resolve these questions. Unfortunately, diagnosing a food allergy is more complicated than that and cannot usually be accomplished with a single simple test.

In Part 2 you will see that the medical history, your description of what your child has experienced, is the most important diagnostic tool. In fact, many families bring tests to our first visit, but I ask them to put aside these results; instead, we discuss what has actually happened to their child. Knowing the key points of the medical history will help your doctor uncover what foods, if any, are responsible for your child's symptoms. I will also discuss how you, your pediatrician, and your allergist can work together to help your child.

The major step in diagnosing food allergy is often found in the details of the history, laboratory tests are helpful to confirm suspicions. When reactions such as anaphylaxis occur suddenly, tests that detect food-specific IgE antibodies, those molecular "antennae" discussed in Chapter 1, are often needed to confirm a diagnosis. Tests used to detect these IgE antibodies include skin prick or scratch and blood tests. You will see how skin and blood tests are used to diagnose a food allergy, and we will explore their limitations. In many situations, to confirm whether a food is tolerated, a doctor must observe your child as he slowly eats the food. This procedure, called an oral food challenge, *will be described in Chapter 11. Next, I consider additional tests you may encounter, some under study and some unproven for diagnosing a food allergy.*

To diagnose a food allergy successfully, it is helpful to understand many of the features of food allergy that were described in Part 1. For example, knowing the foods that most frequently cause problems, knowing the types of illnesses that are caused by a food allergy, and understanding how the body's immune system is responsible for these problems, are prerequisites for interpreting the medical history and selecting and analyzing tests. Of course, the burden of diagnosis rests with your doctor. However, families benefit from knowing what is involved in diagnosing allergies for several practical reasons. Aside from curiosity and enlightenment about your child's food allergies, you will be in a better position to communicate important issues to your doctors to ensure a proper diagnosis. And more important, you will be able to explain to your child why certain tests are done. In Chapter 13, you will meet several of my patients and use what we have learned to diagnose their food allergies.

9 ~ The Medical History

I met 7-year-old Marsha when her parents brought her to me for an evaluation of a possible chicken allergy. She had experienced two rather severe allergic reactions about a month apart. The family explained that her first reaction occurred at a family barbecue when she was eating grilled chicken. Hives, coughing, and lip swelling were treated in the emergency room with several different medications. Her second reaction was quite similar and happened at home during lunch after she had eaten a chicken sandwich. The family was not quite sure what had caused the first reaction and had not discussed the reaction in detail with their pediatrician. Because she had not eaten anything unusual at the time of the first reaction, the family thought that perhaps she was stung by a bee. Her parents brought in a list of allergy tests that were performed by their pediatrician, but I suggested that we talk about the details of Marsha's allergic reactions first.

The Medical History Is More Important Than Tests

A conversation with Marsha's parents provided the most crucial information for making an accurate food allergy diagnosis. Already Marsha's family was quite sure that Marsha had experienced a reaction to chicken because her test for chicken was positive and her tests for insect sting allergy were negative. The testing had been done after there was a second reaction attributed to chicken and the insect sting tests were added because the first reaction was outdoors. However, from what I had already heard, insect stings on both occasions seemed unlikely, and it was uncommon to develop an allergy to chicken at her age. Even though she had tested positive for chicken allergy, we needed to make sure we were not on the wrong track, by assuming that this was a chicken allergy.

When a doctor or allergist considers whether a particular problem can be attributed to a food allergy, many factors come into play. Is the symptom or reaction consistent with an allergic reaction, or is there some other explanation for the symptom? For example, a person can have trouble breathing for different reasons. Food allergy could be one of them, but so could choking, an asthma attack, or pneumonia. Could a food allergy cause the problem that the person experienced? Sometimes reactions from foods are sudden, and when they are, the types of symptoms we expect to see are hives, swelling, trouble breathing, coughing, gastrointestinal problems (such as vomiting) or sometimes poor blood circulation. However, other problems may cause these same symptoms. Sometimes reactions from foods can be chronic, such as itchy hives, atopic dermatitis, or gastrointestinal problems and poor growth. If I am considering food allergy in particular, I will need to know which foods to suspect, when these foods were ingested, and what symptoms developed. Understanding what the doctor may be looking for in a medical history will help you to provide the information to diagnose and treat your child successfully.

Marsha had typical symptoms of an allergic reaction. She experienced coughing, hives, and swelling that responded to antiallergy treatments in the emergency room. If she had rashes that had lasted for days and weeks, I would have considered other causes. For example, a virus could cause coughing and hives. But in this case, her symptoms occurred suddenly, around mealtimes, and fit the symptoms we see in an allergic reaction. Emergency room staff thought she had an insect sting, although she had no pain and no stinger could be found. It seemed appropriate to test for insect sting allergy if no other possible triggers could be determined, but with the second reaction, a food allergy seemed probable, because of the timing and type of symptoms.

What food could have triggered the problem? On both occasions, Marsha had eaten chicken, which would certainly make chicken a likely culprit. However, chicken usually does not cause this type of reaction. In fact, Marsha had eaten chicken throughout her life and even on occasions between the times of the two reactions without incident. With allergies, you would usually expect to have a reaction each time you ate the offending food.

The family seemed convinced that chicken was the common denominator in these two reactions. Even the allergy test was positive for chicken, but I was not convinced. I asked Marsha's family to set aside chicken as the problem. We talked about the first reaction at the barbecue. She had eaten a variety of foods that day. She had ingested various drinks, salads, and snack foods and was running and playing with other children. If that had been her only reaction, I would have been at a loss to find an immediate trigger. I would have assumed that if food was involved, it would probably be a food that she ate infrequently and that was known to cause severe reactions, such as peanuts, tree nuts, fish, or shellfish. However, her regular diet included these foods; besides, she did not eat these foods at the barbecue.

I would have considered nonfood triggers next. For example, had a bee stung her? Had she taken a medication? But she had not taken any medication. Food allergy seemed a likely explanation after the second reaction, and I wanted to know more about the details of her diet on that day. The family had a much better idea of what she had eaten that day because her reaction occurred during lunch. They recalled that she had eaten chicken on wheat bread with lettuce and tomato, carrots, and a glass of milk. But Marsha indicated that her symptoms started after she had eaten yogurt, which her parents had forgotten about. They had focused on chicken because her first reaction developed soon after she had eaten grilled chicken at the barbecue.

Marsha had eaten an orange-flavored yogurt she had never previously eaten that was obtained from a friend's home. What I had therefore learned was that the grilled chicken eaten at the time of the barbecue reaction and the orange-flavored yogurt eaten during the second reaction were the foods ingested closest to the onset of her symptoms. What could grilled chicken and yogurt have in common? I sent the family on a homework assignment to determine how the grilled chicken was prepared and what ingredients were in the orange-flavored yogurt. They returned with a jar of flavoring for grilling chicken and a container of yogurt. The only ingredient that was common to both of these items was annatto. Annatto is a coloring agent derived from a seed and has been reported to cause anaphylactic reactions. It is a common ingredient, but it is also not one that you might frequently encounter. We performed allergy testing for annatto, and, indeed, Marsha had a very strong positive response. Taking the time to consider the medical history enabled us to identify the correct trigger.

Many details, at first glance, may seem unimportant but could be vital to a proper diagnosis. For example, how food is cooked or processed may become an important part of the history. For example, canned tuna and salmon are much less likely to trigger a reaction than fresh fish because the canning process breaks down many of its proteins. Similarly, beans, fruits, beef, and vegetables are more or less allergenic, depending on how they are cooked.

In a medical history, the amount of food that was eaten in relationship to any given reaction is also of interest. For example, sesame may have been tolerated in small amounts on a slice of bread but may have caused a severe reaction when eaten in tahini, a sesame paste. The timing of ingestion of the food in relation to the onset of symptoms is also an important clue for diagnosis. Most reactions would occur minutes after ingesting the food, and it is unusual to have a reaction begin more than an hour afterward, although it is possible. The consistency of reactions is also an important feature. For example, if the food is usually tolerated in meal-sized amounts, it is unlikely the food would suddenly become an allergen.

I also want to know the circumstances surrounding any particular reaction. For example, in the syndrome of food-associated, exercise-induced anaphylaxis, a food that is usually tolerated when eaten without exercise may trigger anaphylaxis if it is eaten followed by exercise. Similarly, a particular ingestion of another food such as alcohol, although usually not an issue for young children, could increase the severity of a reaction because the alcohol may increase the absorption of the food allergen. Aspirin and related medications such as ibuprofen may also increase the likelihood of a reaction for some people. Knowing the circumstances of a reaction is also important because alternate causes may be uncovered. Because Marsha's reaction occurred outdoors, an insect sting allergic reaction needed to be considered.

Detailed Diet Records and Food Labels

If your child has a chronic medical problem, such as frequent vomiting or rashes that come and go, keep diet records. I ask parents to write down everything their child eats during the day and also keep records of symptoms in relation to the various meals that the child ingests. Snacks and everything that goes into your child's mouth should be recorded. Your doctor will be able to analyze records about what foods may be triggering problems, although this is tricky to determine. Save food labels, too, which list potential problem ingredients.

Stacie is a 6-year-old with a cow's milk allergy. Her milk allergy is quite severe, but she did very well for a few years, avoiding milk with only occasional small exposures that resulted in modest reactions. Unfortunately, she did not seem to be outgrowing her allergy. Over a two-month period, Stacie had experienced several allergic reactions to a growing list of foods. She had ingested shrimp on a few occasions, but recently had a sudden allergic reaction to shrimp. She also noticed that soy cheese caused an itchy mouth, even though she had ingested many different soy products without a problem. Even canned tuna fish had recently triggered a reaction even though she tolerated canned tuna fish and other fish prepared fresh. She came to me, therefore, newly avoiding soy, shrimp, and fish.

It is possible to develop a new allergy to foods. This often occurs with peanuts, tree nuts, and seafood, which are foods that are perhaps not eaten very routinely in many people's diet. However, Stacie frequently ate fish and shellfish with no problem, although she had stopped eating them after the two reactions. Soy is an unusual food to become allergic to at her age. I had asked the family to bring in the labels from their food and, indeed, I identified that the soy cheese was a brand that contained cow's milk protein. Her canned tuna fish indicated that it also contained milk protein. With the canned tuna, milk had been used as an additive to keep the fish solid. Stacie was reacting to the milk protein in these products.

The shrimp seemed more of a mystery, and I assumed that she was likely to have developed a shrimp allergy. I performed an allergy test to shrimp, which, surprisingly, was negative. I was still concerned that she might have a shrimp allergy because her reaction to that particular food was a bit more severe, and she had not eaten shrimp for about six months before that reaction. However, the family had indicated that she had continued to eat lobster and crab with no problems. This was interesting because many people with an allergy of significance to one crustacean shellfish will react to others. Delving deeper, I found out the shrimp she had eaten had been frozen originally. We then reviewed the label that did not list milk. A packaging company explained that on occasion the shrimp was processed with milk protein to reduce odor. Stacie had not developed new allergies after all, so there was no need to restrict her diet further.

To help your doctor arrive at a proper diagnosis, write down as much detail as you can about symptoms and keep a careful diet record for at least several days, if chronic problems are involved. Include prescribed and over-the-counter medications on the diet record. Take these with you to doctor visits, so that it may be possible to see any association of certain foods with symptoms. Keeping explicit records of foods eaten around the time of any sudden reactions is also important. If a reaction occurred during a restaurant meal, restaurant personnel may know the ingredients used and even what ingredients were used near the meal during preparation. If the restaurant was using packaged products, they perhaps could provide labels. When you are requesting more information from a store or restaurant, stress that you are not intending to blame the restaurant but that your child's doctor is trying to determine the cause of your child's allergic reaction. These same rules may apply to packaged products if an unexpected reaction occurs. In some cases, the physician may need to intervene when the company is reluctant to disclose proprietary ingredients.

At age 17, Ruben came to my office because of episodes of lip swelling, hives, and breathlessness. The family kept careful diet records for each of these events and had written down minute details of every food he had ingested. One food was common to the four episodes—potato. It is unusual for potato to cause reactions, and Ruben ate potato on many occasions without a problem. I was reluctant to test him for potato because it seemed so unlikely that this would have caused the problem. I asked the family about other possible triggers such as exercise, insect stings, or contact with anything new, but nothing registered. Was Ruben on any medication? No. Did he drink alcohol? No. I interviewed him separately to determine whether there were any other problems or exposures, but there were none.

His symptoms sometimes occurred minutes after a meal, during a meal, or as long as an hour-and-a-half after a meal. Reactions happened at dinnertime meals, after he had returned from wrestling practice. He denied ingesting any snacks or other foods during wrestling. I considered that perhaps some kind of exposure during wrestling might have been a problem, but he wrestled on many other occasions with no symptoms. I asked whether Ruben used any antipain medications for wrestling. On occasion after wrestling, Ruben took ibuprofen for pain, a medication he typically did not use. He was certain, in retrospect, that each of these episodes occurred after he had taken the medication. When I had originally asked whether he was using any medications, he did not mention ibuprofen because it is an over-the-counter medication. However, aspirin sensitivity is a common issue, particularly for triggering asthma, but it is also sometimes associated with more typical allergic reactions such as hives or swelling, which is what he had experienced. Ruben did not have a food allergy, but he was sensitive to aspirin. This turned out to be important information; I gave Ruben specific instructions about avoiding medications that contain aspirin and aspirin-related medications such as ibuprofen.

Before considering allergy testing, tell your doctor all the details that could help with determining whether your child's illness or symptom could be food related, and what the triggering foods could be.

What Your Pediatrician and Allergist Can Do

Your primary care doctor, pediatrician, or family practitioner knows about the many illnesses that children can experience, including allergies and food allergies. Your pediatrician will try to determine whether food allergy is a possible cause of your child's symptoms. In some cases, your pediatrician may suggest testing to confirm an allergy or may suggest a completely different explanation for the problem. Pediatricians care for the many different allergic problems experienced by children such as atopic dermatitis, asthma, allergic rhinitis, anaphylaxis, and food allergies. When a child's diagnosis is unclear, when the allergic problem is complex and can involve a number of explanations, or even when a food allergy is confirmed, your primary care doctor may request consultation with an allergist.

An allergist is specially trained to diagnose and treat all types of allergic disorders, including food allergy. An allergist is initially trained as an internist, a pediatrician, or sometimes both and continues training for two or three additional years to learn more about allergy, immunology, and disorders of the immune system. A board-certified allergist has successfully completed training and has also passed a test indicating competence in the field. Whether an allergist initially trained in internal medicine or pediatrics, allergy training includes the care of both children and adults. Some allergists continue to see all age groups, while others may see just adults or only children. The allergist is trained specifically to obtain a medical history about allergy problems. The allergist performs physical examinations, focusing on allergic problems, conducts allergy tests such as skin tests, and provides expert diagnosis and treatment of allergic disorders, including food allergy. Many details are considered to diagnose and treat food allergy, and the allergist has the tools to provide guidance in this area.

Finding the right allergist for you and your child is similar to finding the right pediatrician. Make sure you have a board-certified allergist. Because your relationship with your allergist is personal, most of the additional issues in finding an allergist to care for your child are personal. I suggest that you ask your pediatrician or family practitioner to recommend allergists. Web sites of professional allergy organizations can be found in Part 9. Some of the professional organization Web sites allow you to enter your zip code and specific problems that your child has been experiencing to find the right fit of an allergist for your child. Finding the right doctor really means finding an individual with whom you feel comfortable. You should expect that a good allergist will take time to listen to the medical history, which is key to diagnosing allergies. Most allergists perform the tests that will be described in Chapters 10 and 11, but in some cases, you may be referred to a specialty center for advanced tests. With the important tools that you have obtained by reading this book, you will be better prepared to work with your primary care doctor and allergist in helping your child. Indeed, the pediatrician or family practice doctor and allergist work together, sometimes with other specialists, such as pulmonologists, dermatologists, or gastroenterologists, to treat various aspects of allergic disease that your child may experience. And when it is time for a doctor's visit, bring along any important medical records, diet records, and a list of questions and concerns.

Diagnosing a food allergy requires carefully considering various points of the medical history. By providing your doctor with details of your child's symptoms and your concerns about their relationship to food, you are well on your way to helping your doctor to arrive at the correct diagnosis. By keeping track of the possible foods that may be involved, collecting detailed information about ingredients, considering the timing of reactions, whether the foods under consideration are ever tolerated, looking at the way that the foods are prepared, and keeping an open mind to various possibilities will help to ensure that the correct tests, if any, are selected and the correct diagnosis is found.

10 ~ Allergy Tests for IgE

Skin and Blood Tests

When a child has a sudden reaction to a food with symptoms such as hives, swelling, or asthma, we would expect to find that his or her body has made IgE antibodies that recognized the food that has caused the reaction. The IgE antibodies are like tiny antennas the immune system has created that sit atop allergy cells, such as mast cells, in various parts of the body. When the food comes in contact with the IgE antibody "antennas" that are able to identify a particular protein, the mast cell is alerted to release chemicals, such as histamine, that cause the various symptoms of an allergic response. These mast cells are distributed in various areas of the body, including the nose, lung, gastrointestinal tract, and skin. One type of allergy test, the allergy prick, or scratch, skin test takes advantage of the fact that mast cells are in the skin, and if they are armed with IgE antibodies to the food your child may be allergic to, we can detect them with simple allergy skin tests. The IgE antibodies also float in the bloodstream as they make their way to various places; they may be captured by mast cells in various areas of the body or by basophils in the bloodstream. Another type of test, a blood test for food-specific IgE antibody, takes advantage of IgE antibodies' ability to be detected while they are floating in the bloodstream. Therefore, both skin tests and blood tests for allergy are measuring the presence of these IgE antibodies. In this chapter, we will explore the details of these two types of tests, how they are conducted, what the results may mean, and the limitations of these tests.

Prick Skin Tests

An allergy prick skin test takes advantage of the fact that there are mast cells throughout the skin that may be armed with a variety of IgE antibody "antennas" capable of detecting proteins your child is allergic to. These IgE antibodies may be directed to allergens that are not related to food, such as animal dander or pollens, but they also may be directed toward the proteins in foods.

Typically, allergy prick skin tests are performed by allergists. The allergists will obtain from a commercial supplier extracts of a variety of foods that can be tested. The manufacturers of these extracts have created diluted samples of various foods. If one places one of these extracts on the skin without scratching the skin's surface, it is very difficult for the food protein to seep in to meet the mast cells. Therefore, small plastic probes with sharp tips are used to scratch or prick the skin so that the food proteins or other allergens reach the mast cells. In some cases, metal probes are used. Some of the devices are made for creating a single scratch at a time, and others, called *multi-testers,* contain eight probes in one plastic piece so that multiple scratches can be made at one time. Because these devices are only scratching the surface of the skin, no bleeding is involved and discomfort is minimal. In some cases, the devices are dipped into the liquid allergen and then scratched onto the skin. In other cases, a drop of the liquid extract is placed on the skin and then the device is pressed through that extract to scratch the surface of the skin. It generally takes ten to fifteen minutes for the food protein to meet the IgE on the surface of the mast cells, to alert the mast cells to release histamine, and for the histamine to leave a bump (wheal) surrounded by a ring of redness (flare). A positive test is itchy and looks like a mosquito bite.

The prick skin test, therefore, represents a quick, accurate, and relatively painless way to detect food-specific IgE antibodies. To prepare for the test, your child would be required to avoid medications such as antihistamines, which can interfere with test results. If your child were taking an antihistamine, then the histamine released from the mast cells during testing would be blocked and would not cause the wheal-and-flare response. Because of this, your allergist would advise you to discontinue your child's antihistamines for a period of time before the tests are performed. Some antihistamines stay in the body for only a short time. Therefore, it may be necessary to avoid certain antihistamines for three or four days before the tests. Other antihistamines may last in the body for a week or two, requiring a longer period of avoidance before testing. Your allergist should provide you with specific instructions on how to avoid these particular medications. Most allergy nose sprays and asthma medications would not affect testing. Some types of depression medications would affect the test results, so discuss this with your doctor.

I generally advise my patients that if discontinuing any of their medications results in disruptive symptoms, then they should not avoid these medications. Instead, we could seek alternatives for testing or alternative medications to keep them comfortable while they are off the antihistamines. Steroid medications would not typically affect the results of these allergy tests if they are taken orally for less than a few weeks. Also, if large amounts of steroids are being placed on the skin where the tests are performed, this may also affect the results. However, steroids inhaled from canisters or nebulizers would not affect the skin test results.

To perform the allergy skin tests, the skin to be tested is typically cleaned with an alcohol wipe. In some cases, the allergist or technician may mark the skin to be tested to be able to identify each test. Two tests are performed to compare with the results of the allergens. One is a saltwater, or saline, control test. No one is allergic to salt water, but some children develop swelling where they are scratched, a reaction called *dermographism.* The allergist must know whether a simple scratch on your child's skin could cause swelling; otherwise, responses to allergens would be interpreted as positive when perhaps the skin simply swelled from being scratched. The allergist will be able to compare the scratch associated with salt water to the allergens being tested.

The other test used routinely for comparison is histamine. In this case, histamine is scratched into the skin and will activate the blood vessels and nerves in the area to cause the wheal-and-flare response and its associated itch. The size of this response to histamine can then be compared with the reactions caused by the food allergens being tested. This test is also important because if your child had taken medications to block the response, such as an antihistamine, then the histamine test would not cause the type of response expected. A typical histamine response has a bump, or wheal, about the size of a pea and a flare that is about the size of a quarter. In some cases, the testing is placed on a child's back. In other cases, they are placed on the arm, between the wrist and elbow, on the same side of the arm as the palm of the hand.

It is possible to do prick skin testing on individuals of any age, including infants. The allergist may need to consider the age of your child in interpreting the tests because an infant may have smaller responses or lack responses in some cases. The location of the test on the body, the age of the child, and the source of the food extracts are all important variables in regard to the types of skin responses that may be seen. For example, testing on the back often results in larger test results than when tests are performed on the arm. There is not a single "correct" location to perform the test because your allergist may decide on a location, depending on the number of tests being performed and the ability of a child to hold still for testing. However, it is important for the allergist to make a note of where the testing was performed so that if tests are compared over time, it is known just how they were done.

Recording the size of the test results can be done in different ways. Some allergists compare the size of the allergen skin test wheal to the size of the skin test wheal of the histamine and saline controls and report this on a scale of 0 to 4 or 5 to indicate the relative size. Others will record each test's size on its own, either on a scale of no response to responses up to 5 or 6 in size, or they may measure the test results and write down the sizes of the wheal and flare in millimeters. Another way of recording the exact results could be to take a picture of the responses or to circle the responses with ink on the skin and then use cellophane tape to transfer the pictures of the circles onto paper that can then be kept in the medical record and also measured.

While the skin-testing procedure is not very painful, there is discomfort associated with it, both during the scratching and during the response when itching might start. Prepare your child for these tests, and work with the allergist or office personnel to help make the procedure as stress-free as possible for your child. When infants are skin-tested, they often show no signs of discomfort during the testing procedure. Much of the stress associated with testing is based on the child's fear and anxiety because of the unusual-looking and foreign procedure. The best tactic to choose to keep your child calm and to make the experience as stress-free as possible depends on your child's personality and temperament. Some families find it helpful to begin discussing the testing procedure in advance of the visit, while others prefer to introduce the issue just before it occurs.

I explain to children that the discomfort is similar to having a fingernail scratch on the surface of the skin. I often demonstrate what this may feel like before actually bringing out the probes and materials used for skin testing. Like any procedure in children, it is helpful to explain each step to avoid surprises. Of course, the manner in which the procedure is explained will depend on the age and developmental level of the child. For younger children, I will usually say the liquid is like a raindrop falling on the skin and that the probe will feel like a fingernail scratch. I also warn them that the area may itch but that they are not allowed to scratch. To undertake this simple procedure with the least amount of fuss and stress, you may need to distract your child in some way. I encourage the person performing the procedure or you, as the parent, to speak continuously with your child during the tests. Singing or reciting during the procedure is a helpful distraction. Counting or saying the alphabet may help. Some families bring portable audio or video devices for the child to listen to if they are not otherwise available in the doctor's office. After the testing is performed, the child may be inclined to scratch, but this would make it difficult to interpret the test results because scratching can inflame the skin. Therefore, your child will be instructed not to scratch the areas, and you will need to help them avoid doing so. Again, distraction is an excellent means to attain this. Young children may play with toys and forget about the slight itch.

Families are often concerned that performing the scratch tests may result in an actual allergic reaction. Indeed, allergens are placed on the skin and scratched onto the surface of the skin to cause localized responses. It is possible that some of these proteins could cause a more wide-ranging allergic reaction. However, studies show that this is extremely rare. The chance of having a severe reaction from skin testing is usually associated with the number of tests performed because if dozens of tests are placed at the same time, there is a higher risk than if just a smaller number are performed. Although the number of tests may vary, depending on the circumstances, it is unlikely that more than a dozen tests will be administered at one time to evaluate food allergies. Some types of allergy tests use a needle to inject an allergen into the skin. This is not advised for food allergy testing because doing so can cause a response that is not relevant to an actual food allergy, and injecting the food also increases the risk of an allergic reaction. Allergy tests are performed in the allergist's office, so that in the rare event of an allergic reaction from prick skin testing, treatments would be immediately available.

Families sometimes ask whether the skin testing itself can cause an allergy in their child. Technically, no studies have specifically evaluated this question. It would be unlikely that a scratch test for a food allergy could cause the allergy because food proteins are common in the environment. People are more likely to be unwittingly exposed to food protein in daily life than from allergy tests. In fact, we often see positive allergy tests in individuals who have had no known exposures to the foods to which they were being tested. In addition, 80 percent of reactions to foods such as peanuts and tree nuts have occurred during what the family considers to be a first-known exposure to the food, even though the immune system must have been exposed to these proteins at some point.

The prick skin test represents a quick, simple, relatively painless way to detect food-specific IgE antibody. It can be performed for any food for any age child. A child undergoing these tests must be off medications that can block the test. Also, the skin must be rash-free in the area where the test will be performed. Proper preparation of your child about the test procedures and using distractions while the test is being performed should help make this a relatively stress-free procedure.

Blood Tests for IgE Antibody

Another way to detect the food-specific IgE antibody "antennas" is to perform a blood test. The blood test is often called a RAST, or RadioAllergo-Sorbent Test. This test used to be performed in the laboratory using radioactivity, but this type of test is no longer done. The name RAST has survived even though the procedure in the laboratory has changed. There are various brands of laboratory tests made by different companies. In each of these tests, results may be reported in a variety of ways. However, the general procedure that these various laboratories are using is the same. They have attached a protein from food to a solid such as a paper disk, plastic bead, or gel matrix. This item is placed in a test tube that contains your child's blood. If IgE antibodies are in the blood, they will attach to the food protein on the paper, plastic, or gel. The test tube is washed so that the components in the blood are removed, leaving just the IgE stuck to the specific food, which is, in turn, attached to the paper, plastic, or gel within the test tube. The test tube is then filled with a protein that can attach to your child's IgE antibody. That protein also contains a molecule that can glow in the dark. By measuring the amount of "glow," the laboratory is able to determine the amount of IgE antibodies for a specific food protein floating in the bloodstream. This procedure has nothing to do with mast cells or histamine, and so it does not matter whether your child has been taking antihistamines or has preexisting rashes, which is an advantage over the skin test. However, one disadvantage of the blood test is that it requires drawing blood.

The fear, pain, and anxiety of a blood test can be addressed in the same way that was described for allergy skin testing, namely, age-appropriate preparation and distraction techniques during the procedure. Topical medications can also be used to numb the surface of the skin, which may make blood drawing easier. However, in my experience, proper mental preparation is most important because general fear and anxiety about the test usually upset the child more than the pain. The blood test is very good at detecting food-specific IgE antibody, but it is, in many circumstances, not quite as good or sensitive as the skin test. A sensitive test is a test that can detect a tiny amount of IgE antibody, and sometimes, but not always, the skin test will be positive when the blood test is negative. The blood test also does not provide an instant answer, as does the skin test, and so your doctor will have to discuss the results on another occasion, usually a number of days after the test has been performed. Last, the blood test is more costly than performing allergy skin tests. As we will see next, the blood tests and skin tests may be used in complementary ways, along with the medical history, for diagnosing a food allergy.

Laboratories may report the results of the blood tests in a variety of units, almost like ounces versus milliliters. Your doctor should keep in mind the type of laboratory test that was performed and the way in which the result was reported when results are compared. Much confusion could occur if different tests or different ways of reporting results are compared without realizing the inconsistencies. For example, results may be reported as counts, percentages, units, classes, or several of these, depending on the manufacturer. Test results from different manufacturers may not be equivalent.

Interpretation of Tests for IgE Antibody

Both the prick skin tests and the allergy blood tests are superb at determining whether your child has produced IgE antibodies to a particular food. However, that is all they can do. *A positive allergy test does not necessarily mean your child will have an allergic reaction if they ingest the food to which they tested positive.* This is a concept that is often difficult to accept but is crucial for understanding how to properly diagnose a food allergy. In studies where families suspect a particular food was a problem, and there were positive allergy tests, only about a third of the children actually reacted to the food to which they tested positive. When skin tests to peanuts were performed randomly in the general population without regard to an allergy history, 5 percent to 8 percent had positive tests. Regarding allergic reactions, we know that 1 percent or fewer of the general population truly has an allergic reaction if they ingest peanuts. Therefore, many people with a positive allergy test can tolerate the food they tested positive to.

What about when the allergy test is negative? If one is evaluating a sudden allergic reaction and the allergy test, in particular the more sensitive prick skin test, for the tested food is negative, there is about a 1-in-20 chance that an allergic reaction will occur. To summarize, a positive allergy test often exists even though a food can be ingested with no problems and a negative allergy test usually, but not always, means that the food will be tolerated. With these types of limitations, you may wonder whether tests are helpful at all! They are incredibly helpful, but they must be interpreted in the context of a medical history.

In addition, the size of an allergy skin test or the amount of IgE antibody detected in a blood test may reflect the chance of having an allergic reaction to the test food. Specifically, the larger the size of the skin test or the higher the amount of IgE to the test food, the greater the likelihood of a clinical reaction.

Studies relating allergy test results to whether a child reacts to a particular food are ongoing. These studies have only addressed a small number of foods, and the results of these studies differ, depending on the ages of the children evaluated and their illnesses. For example, a given test result in an infant, let's say a result of "2," may indicate a very high likelihood that the infant would have an allergic reaction to a food. Yet the same test result of "2" in an older child may not be reflective of a true food allergy. Similarly, a particular test result in a child who has had a sudden allergic reaction to food but does not have atopic dermatitis may have a different meaning than if the same test results were present in a child with atopic dermatitis who has not experienced a sudden allergic reaction to the food.

The diameter of a wheal from a skin test is typically measured in millimeters. When the size of the skin test is about 3 mm, taking into account any correction for dermatographism, the nonspecific swelling of skin from a scratch test, studies have shown that roughly half of the children with this result react to the food. However, when skin tests have wheals of 8 mm, 10 mm, or larger, it is more common to see actual clinical reactions to the foods. However, the exact measurements of the skin test may vary based on techniques the allergists use and, as previously mentioned, the age and medical problems of the child. The general rule is that the larger the skin test, the more likely the child would have an actual allergic reaction caused by the tested food.

Interpreting the blood test is similar, in many ways, to the skin test. Increasing levels of IgE of the tested food would indicate an increased risk of a reaction from eating that food. Some studies have shown that at some particularly high levels of IgE antibody on the blood test, one almost always finds that the child would have a problem with the food. For example, studies of children at about age 5, where roughly half of the children have chronic skin rashes, showed that if the IgE antibody level measured by a particular method called a CAP-RAST (FEIA), which reports its results in kilo International Units per liter (kIU/L), more than 95 percent of children had reactions if their tests were at or above the following levels:

egg	6 kIU/L
milk	14 kIU/L
peanut	15 kIU/L
codfish	20 kIU/L

Studies have also examined soy and wheat allergy in relation to blood test results. A level over 65 kIU/L for soy and 80 kIU/L for wheat was usually associated with allergic reaction but not as strongly as the levels previously shown with the other foods.

Studies have also shown that levels of about 2 kIU/L for egg or milk represented about a 50 percent risk of a reaction in children around 5 years old.

In these various studies, even an undetectable level of IgE (sometimes reported as <0.35 kIU/L) to these foods was sometimes associated with an allergic reaction. In fact, about 10 percent to 30 percent of the children had an allergic reaction to the food, even though their blood test was negative. In most of these circumstances, the skin test would be expected to be positive because it is a slightly more sensitive test. This is an example in which additional information can sometimes be obtained by doing both tests.

In summary, a test may be positive but not always reflect a true clinical allergy. However, a negative test does *not* guarantee there is no allergy. Still, the stronger the result, the more likely there is a true allergy. Of course, these tests are only relevant for illnesses in which IgE antibodies to foods are responsible for the food-allergic reaction.

The studies also indicate that aspects of the medical history and the age of the child may influence the test interpretation. In children who had an unclear history of an allergic reaction to peanuts, half of them tolerated peanuts when their level was less than 5 kIU/L on this particular blood test. However, if a more certain history of an allergic reaction were known, then the level at which half of the children tolerated peanut was 2 kIU/L. For infants around 1-year-old, a level of 2 kIU/L to milk or egg is almost always associated with true allergy to these foods, while the same results in a 5-year-old are associated with true allergy only about half of the time.

I evaluated 6-year-old Eva for the possibility of allergies to eggs, milk, and peanuts. Eva had experienced hay fever symptoms, with itchy, watery eyes and a runny nose for several years, and her pediatrician sent her for a battery of allergy tests to determine what may have been causing her hay fever symptoms. Along with tests for environmental allergens such as dust mites, mold, animal dander, and pollens, her pediatrician sent the CAP-RAST test for egg, milk, and peanut allergies. Her egg level was 0.5 kIU/L, milk was 5 kIU/L, and peanut was 10 kIU/L. Her family was concerned that she may have allergies to these three foods, but the history revealed that she had been eating these foods with no problem throughout her life.

On the basis of studies of children under evaluation for food allergy around Eva's age, she had a 50 percent chance of an allergic reaction to egg, more than a 50 percent chance of an allergic reaction to milk, and more than a 90 percent chance of an allergic reaction to peanuts. However, Eva had been eating these foods with no signs of a problem throughout her entire life. I would have had no clear-cut reason to suspect that eggs, milk, or peanuts were causing seasonal hay fever symptoms, and I would not have performed tests to these particular foods in the first place. I explained to Eva's family that it is possible for the body's immune system to make antibodies to certain foods and yet a child could tolerate them. If Eva had some type of allergy symptom after ingesting one of the foods, I might be interpreting these exact same numbers differently. I suggested that she continue to ingest these foods, which made the family concerned that she might someday have an allergic reaction. I further explained that, although it is possible to develop an allergic reaction to any food at any time in your life, it would not be my recommendation to stop eating the food that has already been tolerated. In fact, there are some studies showing that doing so could be detrimental and associated with later problems, such as allergies to that food.

It is easy for doctors and families to focus on test results. It is useful and convenient to know that some studies show that particular allergy test results may be highly related to clinical reactions in children in those studies. However, the clinical history must not be ignored when these tests are being interpreted.

Using Allergy Tests to Track a Food Allergy over Time

One useful aspect of allergy test results is that they can be followed over time. When a child is outgrowing a food allergy, we will typically see that the tests will remain the same or decrease over time. If the child is not outgrowing the food allergy, we may see that the tests are increasing over time or remaining the same but at a level where allergic reactions are still common. Families often ask why an allergy test would increase even though their child has not been eating the food. This occurs frequently, but we do not know exactly why. The body's production of IgE antibody naturally increases as a child gets older. Therefore, a level of, say, 2 kIU/L in a 1-year-old may be

IN DEPTH ON DIAGNOSTIC TESTING

Why might a child be able to tolerate the food with no problem if the IgE antibody test is positive? Why is it that a child may outgrow a food allergy but continue to have a positive test result? Why is it that a test may be negative, but an individual would still react to a food? Answers to these questions are not definitive; however, studies offer possible explanations.

When an allergy test is performed, whether it is a skin test or a blood test, we are measuring the ability of an IgE antibody to contact and attach to a food protein. However, a blood test or skin test is different than ingesting a food. When a food is eaten, it goes to the digestive system, and the proteins in the food may become altered. Recall that protein is the part of the food that is involved in allergic responses. Proteins are composed of a chain of amino acids like a chain of beads on a baby bracelet that spell out words. The IgE antibodies detect the words and segments of words. When you ingest the food, these "bracelets" may be changed in shape or chopped into smaller pieces. An allergy skin test or blood test could be positive even though the food can be eaten with no problems because the digestive system has modified the protein so that it becomes less likely to be seen by the IgE once the protein is digested. The unaltered protein is "seen" when the scratch test or blood test is used, but the digested protein has become "invisible" so the food is tolerated when eaten.

Another reason that a test may be positive even though the food is tolerated is that the test may be detecting certain proteins in the food that look similar among related foods or other proteins in nature. If the cross-reactive proteins are not potent allergens, usually easily digested proteins are not potent allergens, the positive tests may not be important. For example, an individual who is allergic to peanuts—a bean—may have tests that are positive for a variety of beans that share the similar-looking proteins. Usually a person would not react to these other beans, such as peas or string beans, even though they may have an allergic reaction to peanut. In this example, there are some proteins that the immune system can see in these beans (a positive test), but the proteins that are seen are not ones that are likely to trigger an allergic reaction when they are eaten. However, the more potent allergen in peanut is the one causing the reactions. Similarly, your child might react to proteins in pollens that resemble proteins in a variety of fruits or vegetables. Therefore, tests of related foods may be positive, for example, a positive test for apple in a child with a birch pollen allergy, but the proteins are not strong allergens; they are destroyed by heat and digestion and usually do not cause reactions. However, the tests will often be positive even though the food is tolerated when eaten.

Individuals who have atopic dermatitis often make IgE antibody for numerous items in the environment and will frequently have positive tests to numerous foods or other allergens, but they may not always have illnesses associated with exposures to these proteins. In a sense, the immune system is making background "noise" by attacking many items in the environment and in foods. Doctors must acknowledge this tendency when interpreting tests in children whose immune systems generally make a large amount of IgE antibodies.

In all of these circumstances, the tests are very good at identifying that your child's body has made an IgE antibody, but they miss the real-life situation of exposures by ingesting the food in the context of a meal.

In some cases, a test is negative and yet a child reacts when the food is consumed. One explanation for this circumstance is that the allergic reaction has nothing to do with the production of IgE antibodies. As discussed in Chapters 1 and 4, certain illnesses, including atopic dermatitis and a variety of gastrointestinal allergies, may be caused by parts of the immune system that do not involve IgE antibodies. In these situations, a negative test is expected. However, there may also be circumstances where a test is negative even though a reaction is sudden and a positive test is expected. In some circumstances, a very low production of IgE may be hard to detect or that there could be a localized production of IgE, for example, in the intestines, resulting in immediate reactions without being able to detect IgE to the food through skin or blood tests.

Another possibility to explain a negative test despite a true allergy is that what is being used in the test is not appropriate. For example, an individual may have an itchy mouth from ingesting an apple and yet a test with apple extract is negative. The problem here is that fresh apple was causing the allergic reaction, but the test used a commercial extract, wherein the apple protein may have degraded with time, a process like digestion or cooking, and become more like cooked apple, a tolerated food. Individuals who react to raw apple or other raw fruits or vegetables often tolerate that food when it is cooked; therefore, a commercial skin test extract may not reflect the situation correctly. In these circumstances, your allergist may use a homemade extract; for example, the juice from a fresh apple, pricked onto the skin to determine whether there is a positive test associated with the history of symptoms with raw apple or other raw fruits or vegetables.

In summary, a test may be positive or negative and not corroborate what has been observed in your child's experiences with eating certain foods. Although it may be disheartening to know that a positive or a negative test does not always diagnose or exclude an allergy, these tests, when interpreted by individuals who consider the history and features of food allergy, are helpful for diagnosing your child. With greater understanding of the tests, features, and limitations, you will appreciate how your doctor can use these tests to your child's advantage and that a diagnosis is more than a test result.

equivalent to a higher level, for example, 10 kIU/L in a 5-year-old. In this sense, rising test levels over time may not mean that circumstances are any worse but, rather, that the allergy has not been outgrown.

Families are sometimes concerned that their child is experiencing exposure that may be causing the test results to increase. No studies have specifically addressed this concern. However, in our experiences of doing oral food challenges, a procedure where the food is purposefully given to a child who may or may not be allergic to it, we have not seen increases in allergy test results following this procedure. However, exposure to the food during a doctor-supervised feeding is perhaps different than exposures from accidental ingestions of the food because the doctor administers the food gradually and stops at the first sign of trouble. I would not expect a family has caused their child's IgE level to rise through accidental exposure because we see elevated test results in individuals where there has been no convincing evidence or knowledge of accidental exposures.

Interpretation of Tests for Chronic Illness Caused by Food Allergy

Doug is an 11-month-old infant who came to my office to be evaluated for the role of food allergies or other allergies in his severe atopic dermatitis. A detailed dietary history indicated that he was ingesting a milk-based formula and several fruits, grains, and vegetables. The family also had a cat in their home. The family had suspected that apples, peaches, and banana may have caused Doug's allergic symptoms. The specific symptom was an increase in eczema. Doug had not been exposed to several foods, including peanuts and fish. Doug was already using an excellent regimen of skin care but was still experiencing significant discomfort. Therefore, his family wanted to find out what was triggering his eczema.

Although I knew that apple, peach, and banana were unlikely causes of Doug's allergic reactions, the family's history was somewhat convincing, and I was eager to test these foods. But I was also suspicious of foods that were part of his diet and known to be associated with food-allergic reactions, such as egg, milk, wheat, and soy. I performed skin tests to the common food allergens, including peanut, a food he had not yet eaten, because the family was concerned about adding it to his diet. Cat allergen, also a potential trigger for itchy skin, was also tested.

The tests were positive for milk, egg, wheat, soy, peanut, apple, and cat but negative for peach and banana. A negative test usually means the food can be tolerated and because peach and banana are unlikely to cause a problem for children with atopic dermatitis, I thought these could remain in the diet. Apple is also not likely to cause increased eczema, but with the large skin test, I would consider further whether it was an issue because the family suspected it. Cats would need to be avoided.

I performed blood tests to get a better idea about the likelihood of a reaction to eggs, milk, wheat, soy, and peanuts. The blood test result was negative for apple, but the skin test is better for detecting IgE antibody than the blood test, so this was not an unusual result. Some of the test results were in ranges where studies showed that virtually 95 percent or more of the children are truly allergic, and this included a level of 20 kIU/L to egg and 45 kIU/L to peanut. Because of the combination of generous skin tests and higher blood-test results, I recommended that Doug avoid these foods.

The results were less definitive for several other foods. The wheat skin test had been positive, and the blood level was 5 kIU/L, which is in a range where most children tolerate wheat. I suggested that Doug could continue to have wheat in his diet because the family had not suspected wheat, and the skin test was only a modest size, while the blood test was low. The story was different for soy. He had both a positive skin test and a level to soy of 30 units on the blood test, which, together, I interpreted as a 30 percent or 40 percent risk of soy allergy. Even though I was not sure whether he had a soy allergy, I suggested, for now, that the family eliminate soy from Doug's diet. Finally, his milk tests showed a level of 3 units, which is in a range where children like Doug have about a 50 percent risk of a reaction to milk. I recommended he avoid milk. Happily, Doug's skin improved about 80 percent on elimination of these several foods. However, I was ultimately not certain whether he was truly allergic to milk, soy, or apple, and further testing would need to be performed to find out whether these were truly a problem. This additional testing, the oral food challenge, will be discussed in Chapter 11. To evaluate the role of food in chronic conditions, such as atopic dermatitis, allergy testing is often an excellent guide, but a food-elimination diet and doctor-supervised oral food challenges may be needed to confirm the results.

Severity of a Reaction

A common misconception about interpreting allergy tests is that they reflect severity. Imagine two children who have peanut allergy sitting next to each other. One child has a peanut skin test of 5 mm and a blood level of 5 kIU/L, while the other child has a skin test that is twice that size and an IgE antibody level of 50 kIU/L, ten times that amount. You might expect that the child with the larger skin test and a higher IgE to peanut in a blood test would have more severe reactions to peanut and perhaps react to smaller amounts of ingested peanut. However, this is not the case. It is quite possible that the child with the smaller test results or lower levels would have the more severe reaction. The severity of a reaction depends on many factors, including the general health of the child, whether the child has asthma, and how much food was eaten. Most studies have not shown a direct relationship of the test result with severity. Furthermore, reactions often vary from time to time, also based on numerous factors apart from the test results. If your child's test result has increased over time, this would indicate, unfortunately, that perhaps the allergy has not been outgrown, but it would not necessarily mean the reactions would have become more severe.

Trusting the Test Results

A doctor must always consider whether a test result is accurate. A family asked me to evaluate their 4-year-old child, who had experienced what appeared to be two significant allergic reactions to ingestion of peanut butter. The medical history revealed no alternative explanation for the reactions other than peanut had caused these responses. Both skin tests and blood tests had been negative, but because the reactions seemed so convincing and apparently associated with peanut, I did not dismiss the story and performed an oral food challenge; I observed him eat peanut under controlled circumstances. He had a reaction. This is an extremely rare event, but it indicates that tests are not always perfect and that the medical history must never be ignored.

Skin tests and blood tests for IgE antibodies to foods are excellent for identifying a possible allergy, but they do not make a diagnosis. Individuals with positive tests may not react to the foods. Additional predictive information is obtainable from the size of the skin tests or the level of IgE on the blood test, although there have not been studies thus far to consider all foods in all circumstances of age and disease. Specifically, predictive information from studies has primarily focused on eggs, milk, peanuts, and codfish regarding skin test size or blood level and their relationship to outcomes. The interpretation of a particular test result may vary by the age of the child and the type of illness. A negative test is a good sign that there will not be a sudden type of reaction, but it is not a guarantee and must be interpreted in the context of the medical history. The test levels do not, in a simple way, reflect severity of a reaction. While selection and interpretation of the tests must be guided by the medical history, in some cases, the tests and information from the history provide a definitive diagnosis. However, in some cases, the test results and history do not provide a definitive diagnosis, and it may be unclear whether the food is really problematic. An unclear diagnosis may require further testing, such as doctor-supervised ingestion of the food.

11 ~ Elimination Diets and Oral Food Challenges

When a child has almost daily symptoms of skin rashes or gastrointestinal symptoms that may be attributable to foods, and the test results are equivocal or irrelevant to the underlying reason for the illness, then it often becomes necessary to perform trial elimination diets to see whether the chronic symptoms improve or disappear. Usually, knowledge about the common triggering foods, and the results of some tests, will help with devising a diet free of problematic foods. Depending on the problem, it is usually necessary to stay on this elimination diet for days to weeks to see whether symptoms resolve. If the symptoms improve on an elimination diet, the next obvious question is: Which of the foods removed from the diet might have been the problem food(s)? Adding foods back to the diet, a procedure usually done under medical supervision, is called an *oral food challenge*. An oral food challenge is the most definitive way to diagnose a food allergy. If an individual tolerates ingesting a food without symptoms, it may be concluded that he or she is not allergic to the food. An oral food challenge can be used to diagnose essentially any problem attributed to food, even nonallergic adverse reactions to foods. The oral food challenge is a way of determining whether someone is reactive to a food when the allergy tests and history do not strongly indicate an allergy.

Elimination Diets

Twelve-year-old Zachary had experienced years of discomfort with swallowing. On several occasions, food had become stuck in his throat, and he also experienced vomiting and poor weight gain. He was eventually evaluated by a gastroenterologist who performed an endoscopy and biopsy of his esophagus. During that procedure, a tube was placed into his throat and into the esophagus, which connects the mouth and stomach. The gastroenterologist determined that many eosinophils were in Zachary's esophagus and therefore diagnosed *eosinophilic esophagitis.* Eosinophilic esophagitis is considered to be a response to foods for many people who have this disorder (see Chapter 4). Therefore, allergy testing was undertaken. I found that Zachary had positive tests to egg, chicken, and seven other foods. However, he had negative allergy tests to several common allergenic foods that are associated with this disorder. Specifically, his tests were negative for milk, wheat, and soy. In this disorder, allergy tests for IgE antibody are not very accurate in determining which foods may or may not cause symptoms. To best determine whether foods were triggering Zachary's illness, and in an attempt to identify the specific problematic foods, we embarked on an elimination diet.

Zachary's medical history revealed that as an infant he had problems with reflux attributed to milk. To move forward with an elimination diet, I took a careful history of what Zachary currently enjoyed eating, and, indeed, he had a varied diet. I explained three types of elimination diets to Zachary and his family. In the first type, specific foods would be selected to be removed from his diet. For example, he might avoid the foods to which he tested positive. The family and Zachary would be careful to read labels and prepare fresh foods that lacked the specific list of nine items to which he tested positive. However, in this particular disorder, it is not very likely that we would have identified all of the causal foods based only on the positive allergy skin tests.

In the second type of elimination diet, I would prescribe exactly what Zachary would be allowed to ingest. In this diet, I would eliminate all common allergens, such as milk, egg, wheat, soy, peanuts, nuts, and seafood, and I would also eliminate certain foods known to commonly be problematic for individuals with eosinophilic esophagitis. This would include a rice- or a corn-based diet but not both and one type of meat instead of several. Zachary would be limited to heated versions of certain fruits and vegetables because cooking destroys some of the potentially allergenic proteins in these foods. While this is a very narrow diet, it would allow him to have a nutritious diet for six or eight weeks, during which time we would see how his symptoms responded. However, there would be a risk that a problem food remained in the diet. The third diet is an *elemental diet.* In this type of diet, anything that could be problematic would be excluded. This type of diet requires a nutritionally balanced formula. Amino acid–based formulas, unlike cow's milk–based or soy-based formulas, constitute the building blocks of proteins—amino acids—so it is impossible to have an allergic reaction to this type of formula. While there are other constituents of these amino acid–based formulas, there has not been any widespread report of allergic reactions to them. We would generally select perhaps one or two additional foods to go along with the elemental diet.

Zachary was not very excited about the elemental diet; however, this would be the most definitive way to see whether diet changes alone could resolve the problem. If allergy symptoms lessened, then several foods at a time would be added back to the diet; we would look for symptoms and possibly do additional biopsies. After several discussions with the family, we composed a diet for Zachary that was a prescribed "eat only these foods" diet where he received a list of foods that we hoped would be "safe" foods. Zachary determined what he was or was not willing to eat. He approved only food he'd feel comfortable eating for a number of weeks. He also met with a dietitian to ensure that this diet was nutritionally balanced. Even though he tested negative to several of the major allergens, these were also removed from his diet. If his symptoms diminished on this diet, he would undergo another endoscopy and biopsy to see whether the inflammation had reduced. If he was better, we would gradually add more foods to his diet in groups of three or four foods at a time, saving the higher-risk foods for last.

Zachary followed this diet and experienced resolution of his symptoms. A repeat biopsy showed almost complete clearing of the allergic inflammation in his esophagus, and over the subsequent months we were able, by trial and error, to add a variety of foods back into his diet. His final diet excluded seven foods that seemed to be problematic, including milk.

As evidenced for Zachary, elimination diets are useful in determining whether chronic problems such as intestinal problems, chronic skin rashes, or other chronic disorders that may be food related respond to dietary changes.

When it is known that a particular food causes a problem for a child, eliminating that food from the diet is not a trial elimination diet. Elimination of a known food allergen is *treatment* of a food allergy and would be undertaken as such. Selection of the foods to be eliminated from the diet depends on the disorder, the history, and the test results. When test results are positive to a particular food and the potential remains for that food to cause an immediate or dangerous type of allergic reaction, then that food would not be added back to the diet at home but would be added back under direct physician supervision in a procedure called an *oral food challenge.*

Oral Food Challenges

I had been evaluating 3-year-old Sharon since she was 11 months old, a time when she experienced hives following ingestion of milk. She had been breast-fed and then was fed a soy formula. But when she was given a taste of milk at 11 months, she developed the allergic reaction. The family brought her to me for an evaluation around that time; she had a skin test the size of 3 mm and a blood test result of 3 kIU/L. For an 11-month-old girl, those tests are highly predictive of an allergic reaction to milk, and considering that she had symptoms shortly after ingesting milk, I diagnosed a cow's milk allergy. I evaluated Sharon again at age 2. She had been doing well except once when she licked ice cream and then cried for a while; lip swelling may have occurred. Her allergy skin test at that time was 5 mm, and her blood level was 9 kIU/L. Those particular results at that age, and her reaction to ice cream, indicated that she had more than a 90 percent chance of milk allergy. When she saw me on her next visit, she was 3 years old, and she had not experienced any allergic reactions during the preceding year. Her sibling had indicated that she may have taken a bite of a chocolate chip cookie with no reaction. Her skin test was 3 mm and the blood level was 2 kIU/L. Considering that she may have had a small accidental exposure to milk with no problem, and the current test results, I estimated that she had about a 50 percent chance of tolerating milk. Over the two years that I had known Sharon, she had mild atopic dermatitis, and she had not experienced any episodes of asthma. She was otherwise on a generally unrestricted diet, although she had not tried peanuts, but her peanut test was negative. To know whether Sharon was truly still allergic to milk, she would need an oral food challenge.

An oral food challenge is performed to determine definitively whether a food is tolerated. Although Sharon had an IgE-antibody-mediated food allergy, the oral food challenge can be performed for any type of underlying reason for an adverse response to food, allergic or not, or whether IgE antibody mediated or not. The food is given in gradually increasing amounts from very tiny amounts to amounts that usually trigger allergic responses in people who are sensitive. We also ensure that a child can tolerate a meal-sized serving of the food before allowing the food to be eaten as a regular part of the diet.

In an oral food challenge, the food could be provided to the child without disguising it in any form, for example, a child allergic to milk would drink a glass of milk or eat ice cream. This is called an *open food challenge,* and it is a simple procedure to perform because the natural form of the food is being used. However, this type of challenge is open to bias because the child and the family will know that a possible allergen is being ingested. When there is a potential for bias, it is possible for a child to report subjective adverse feelings such as mouth symptoms or stomach symptoms. It is also possible for parents and for physicians to have additional nervousness with any type of symptom that may develop because they know the potential allergen is being eaten. However, this is the simplest form of an oral food challenge. If the food is tolerated, this would indicate that there is no problem, and the food could be added to the diet.

A food challenge can be devised to hide the food to minimize bias as a child's reactions are evaluated. One way is to hide the food to be tested in another food. For example, milk powder may be mixed into applesauce. Egg powder can be mixed into fruit juices, applesauce, or potato. It may take a lot of creativity to hide one food in another food, but this can be accomplished. In some cases, the food may be hidden in opaque capsules that would be swallowed, but this procedure is generally reserved for adults. When a food is given in a hidden form, but the doctor or health care specialist knows that the food is in the tested substance, the procedure is called a *single-blind oral food challenge.* In single-blind food challenges, bias may be reduced for the child or parent, but the doctor or nurse observing the food challenge may have additional biases and may consider that a reaction is occurring when perhaps it is not. Therefore, the surest way to perform an oral food challenge that eliminates bias is called a *double-blind, placebo-controlled oral food challenge* (DBPCFC).

In the DBPCFC, the food to be tested is hidden; another feeding will not contain the food to be tested, but it will look, taste, and smell the same as the tested food. A third party, who will not be observing the feeding, prepares the food. This person would also randomly determine the order in which the feeding would be given. For example, the child would slowly ingest a food that may or may not have the tested food hidden in it in the morning, and if there is no problem, they would ingest the same feeding in the afternoon. It would not be known to the physician watching the feeding or to the parents or child which of those two feedings contained the tested food. Both of these supervised feedings would have been given in increasing amounts to determine whether symptoms occurred. If both of those feedings were tolerated, then a larger, meal-sized portion would be eaten before the tested food was allowed back into the diet.

The time the food is given can be adjusted, depending on the history of previous reactions. Sharon had an immediate reaction to milk, but in some disorders, such as intestinal disorders or rashes, reactions may occur hours or sometimes days after the food is ingested. The oral food challenges can be adjusted to allow for dosing over longer periods of time and for longer periods of observation.

The DBPCFC is time consuming and labor intensive, and it is usually reserved for situations where an individual had an unclear or ambiguous reaction to an open or single-blind challenge, for research studies, or for situations where a doctor believes a panic, or fear, response from the procedure may occur if the child knew when they were eating the food. For Sharon, who had never experienced fear about eating and had always had clear-cut symptoms from an exposure to milk, I thought it was appropriate to offer an open or a single-blind challenge. Her parents were concerned that she might not immediately enjoy the taste of milk products because she had been kept away from them for so long. They thought hiding the milk in another item made sense; however, they were still uncertain whether they wanted to undertake this food challenge. They were concerned about Sharon having a reaction.

Deciding Whether to Undertake an Oral Food Challenge

Many issues need to be considered before undertaking a food challenge. Risk is a major concern. An oral food challenge can result in an allergic reaction that can have mild or severe symptoms. By starting with very small amounts and gradually increasing to meal-sized amounts, we reduce the risk of triggering a severe allergic reaction. For Sharon, we are not going to fill her stomach with a large amount of something to which she may be allergic. If the test results or Sharon's history indicated a high likelihood of allergy, I would be uncomfortable offering the food challenge. If I had estimated, for example, a 90 percent chance of reacting to milk and Sharon's family still wanted to go ahead with the food challenge, I would not be in favor of that, and I would explain that her odds of tolerating milk would improve with age. However, under some circumstances, I might allow someone with a high risk of reaction to undergo a food challenge. For example, if Sharon had been avoiding milk, was 14 years old, and still had a 10 percent chance of tolerating milk, that small change would look much better because at that age it would no longer be likely for her chances to change much with time. And if she passed the challenge, her diet restrictions would be over.

However, Sharon was only 3 years old, and the 50-50 chance she might tolerate the food made the decision difficult for her family to make. If Sharon had to avoid numerous foods and nutritional issues were involved,

I would have supported a food challenge, even if the odds were not that good because adding additional foods would allow better growth. Sharon followed an otherwise unrestricted diet and was having no nutritional issues. The final issue for Sharon had to do with expanding her diet with age-appropriate foods and essentially declaring that she had no further food allergies. Again this was a personal decision for her family.

The family was also concerned whether eating the food at this point would affect Sharon's tolerance for the food in the event she had a positive reaction. That was difficult to answer because not many studies have focused on this. However, in one study our research group conducted, a physician-supervised oral food challenge did not seem to exacerbate an allergy. In fact, most children eventually tolerate a food, even though we may be performing yearly oral food challenges with that food.

Sharon's family was concerned about the safety of an oral food challenge. They favored the oral food challenge because, if she passed, it would mean Sharon and her family would no longer worry about food. But they wanted me to assure them that the food challenge would be safe. I explained the safeguards we would follow. First, I assess the risk of the challenge. Depending on a child's past history of reactions, whether she has asthma (asthma is a risk factor for a severe reaction), and her profile of allergy tests, I decide whether the food challenge would likely trigger a severe reaction. Although any feeding may result in a severe reaction, I am considering many issues at once to determine a likely outcome: Would Sharon react and, if she did, would she have a severe reaction?

No deaths have been reported from physician-supervised oral food challenges. However, only physicians and personnel familiar with treating anaphylaxis and with performing these challenges should conduct them. Allergists sometimes oversee challenges at specialty centers and hospitals.

In any food challenge, we start with small quantities of the food and gradually increase doses by serving larger portions over ten- to fifteen-minute intervals, so we can stop the challenge if signs of a reaction appear without overloading the stomach. If I thought that Sharon was at high risk for a reaction, I might space the doses out further or use even smaller doses. Medications and personnel are available to identify and treat an allergic reaction. Decisions about the possible severity of a reaction during an oral food challenge can also affect where the challenge is performed. For a lower risk of reaction, the procedure may be performed in a doctor's office. For riskier oral food challenge, a hospital may be appropriate. The possible risk of a reaction may affect whether an intravenous (IV) should be inserted before the procedure begins. An IV could be used to administer certain medications or fluids.

Sharon's tests indicated a 50-50 chance of a reaction, but she did not have asthma or any severe prior reactions. If she did react, it would probably not be severe. I decided to perform the oral food challenge in a hospital. Sometimes I will insert an IV ahead of time if I think that there is a likelihood that we would need to administer medications or fluids for a severe reaction. This was unnecessary for Sharon; however, if a severe reaction occurred, an IV could be placed during the reaction.

Her parents asked whether Sharon could have a recurrence of allergies to a food she was able to eat during the test. This was an excellent question. We have not seen a recurrence of allergies to foods such as milk, egg, wheat, or soy once an individual passes an oral food challenge. However, my research group was the first to report that children could develop a recurrence of a peanut allergy. Children with a recurrence of peanut allergy typically had avoided peanut for a long time after they tolerated it during their oral food challenge. The specific issues regarding the long-term course of food allergies are described in detail in Chapter 28. I advise performing oral food challenge to foods only when it is highly likely that that food will be incorporated into the diet afterward.

If Sharon did not pass the oral food challenge, her family asked, would her symptoms indicate future reactions? That is, if she had a mild reaction from the milk during the challenge, would all of her future reactions also be mild? Reactions to foods may be similar from time to time, but the severity of a particular reaction is also unpredictable. Therefore, it would not be a good idea to undertake an oral food challenge simply to see what types of symptoms a child may experience because they may be more or less severe on future occasions. Given all of this information, Sharon's family decided to proceed with the oral food challenge.

Preparing for an Oral Food Challenge

To prepare a child to undertake an oral food challenge, it is important to explain the procedure in advance. Your child will be asked to ingest the food gradually. The child begins the food challenge on an empty stomach and may be allowed to have a drink of water or juice up to about two hours before the procedure. We will typically schedule the procedure in the morning so that the empty stomach is not uncomfortable. Most children have been avoiding the food for a while. However, if the food is being evaluated because of a chronic disease, such as atopic dermatitis, we would have them strictly avoid the food at least two weeks before undertaking the food challenge. For young children, cooperation is certainly an issue, and I discussed with the family in advance the types of foods that Sharon enjoyed eating. I had prepared in advance a potato pancake and also applesauce that contained milk protein because those were two of Sharon's favorite foods. Sharon was going to undergo a single-blind food challenge because we were not sure whether she would have an adverse feeling from ingesting straight milk or ice cream.

Sharon was also a picky eater, and we had the family bring in her favorite plates, bowls, and utensils. We also had a television with some of Sharon's favorite DVD movies. Sharon was not in the mood to try the potato pancake, but she was happy to eat the applesauce. Over a period of an hour and fifteen minutes, she ingested applesauce with the equivalent of three ounces of milk hidden in it in powder form. Before the oral food challenge was started and before each new dose, Sharon's skin, breathing, and behavior were reviewed. Some symptoms are subtle. Some children will become less playful or less active if they start to feel ill during a food challenge. Other subtle symptoms include children scratching at their mouths or making clucking tongue sounds to relieve an itchy mouth. On rare occasions, the symptoms are not very clear-cut, and the result of the oral food challenge may remain uncertain; if this occurs, the procedure can be repeated at another time. The obvious symptoms are hives, vomiting, or other symptoms of an anaphylactic reaction. I had on hand all types of medications used to treat an allergic reaction. Should Sharon have developed any symptoms, we would have stopped giving her the food and treated her appropriately. We were also prepared for an anaphylactic reaction.

Emotional issues are involved in undertaking an oral food challenge, and a discussion among the physician, parents, and child must consider the age and temperament of the child. Whether to perform the oral food challenge also should be considered in the context of these emotional components. Sharon had no specific fear of food, but some children refuse food after they have experienced adverse events. There is always a risk that if a reaction should occur during the feeding, this may cause additional anxiety for a child. Most children do well even after they have had a reaction to a food during an oral food challenge. Explain to your child that she is eating the food under medical supervision to see whether the food can be tolerated; do not promise that she will be able to tolerate the food when the procedure starts. If a reaction occurs, we stress that the child's family will help her avoid the food to stay healthy and safe.

Families are usually in tune with whether their child would be able to undertake the procedure easily. You can help by giving the doctor or the nurses involved "inside information" about your child. Perhaps your child prefers certain games or food prepared a special way. Advise the medical staff about these issues. For example, one of my patients underwent a blind oral food challenge for corn. Corn protein was hidden in potatoes, but he refused it. Corn protein was hidden in four other food he usually enjoyed, but he would just lick the food and refuse to open his mouth to eat it. We finally decided to make corn pasta, but he would not eat this, even though he ate rice pasta with no problem. We continued to try several other varieties of food and this 5-year-old boy would indicate that he was willing to try each new type, but when it came time to eat it, he refused. We finally exhausted all possibilities to give him the food when he declared that he knew we were trying to feed him corn, and he knew that he was not supposed to eat corn. That was the reason he was refusing it. This is an example of the importance of explaining the procedure in detail to a child and having them understand why they are being tested.

Sharon tolerated the entire blinded challenge, but we wanted to ensure that she could consume a meal-sized portion of milk before letting her add milk to her diet. Various studies have shown that approximately 3 percent of the time, although an individual tolerated a modest amount during a blinded food challenge, they still reacted to a larger amount of the food prepared in its usual way. As she watched cartoons, Sharon was fed two scoops of vanilla ice cream. She seemed to enjoy it and had no symptoms. Sharon has now added milk to her diet.

As the family was preparing to leave, they asked if they needed to continue to carry self-injectable epinephrine for Sharon. While it was highly unlikely that Sharon would develop any further symptoms since she tolerated a meal-sized feeding of milk, I often suggest to families that they continue to have a self-injectable epinephrine available for about a year after a food challenge and with successful and regular incorporation of the food into the diet. Aside from the issues mentioned previously about recurrence of peanut allergy, it is not likely that Sharon would redevelop a milk allergy. However, to reduce anxiety and for comfort, it may be helpful to continue to have emergency medication available until everyone is comfortable that the food is tolerated without a problem, assuming the child has no other allergies. Because of the experience of recurrence of peanut allergy, I recommend emergency medications for peanut allergy be kept on hand a year or two, assuming peanut has become a regular part of the diet.

Sometimes, in the excitement of a child's passing an oral food challenge and being able to add a food to the diet, parents may not realize that the new foods and products available to them may have other allergens. If Sharon had a soy allergy, then she would need to avoid milk products that contained soy, for example. Labels still need to be read carefully as the diet is expanded.

When a food challenge is unsuccessful and a reaction occurs, disappointment is unavoidable. However, I emphasize to families that their efforts to avoid the food are for a good reason because the child is allergic. Also, many families find comfort in seeing their child's allergic reactions, which gives them the confidence to recognize and treat future reactions.

~

Elimination diets are often followed by reintroducing foods through doctor-supervised oral food challenges; and oral food challenges performed when tests and history are not definitive for a diagnosis are the surest way of determining whether a food is tolerated. Oral food challenge is generally a safe and a definitive procedure to determine whether a food can be added to the diet.

12 ~ Other Tests

There are limitations on our ability to make a simple, definitive diagnosis of food allergy. Allergy tests for IgE antibodies are far from perfect, certain food allergies are not associated with IgE at all, and oral food challenges carry risks of triggering an allergic reaction. Therefore, additional ways of testing for a food allergy have been investigated. Some of the improved types of food allergy tests will be discussed in Chapter 30. Here we will explore one type of test, termed the *atopy patch test,* which has seen investigated as a way to detect non-IgE-mediated food allergies. We will also consider tests that remain in use but are considered "unproven and experimental" by professional allergy organizations.

Use of Patch Tests for Non-IgE-Mediated Food Allergy

Sudden allergic reactions with symptoms such as hives, asthma, or vomiting are expected to be associated with positive tests for IgE antibody, that is, positive skin prick tests or positive blood tests. However, several food-allergic disorders, most of them with chronic symptoms, are either never or only rarely associated with a positive allergy skin test or blood test. Examples of these illnesses are food protein-induced enterocolitis syndrome, enteropathy syndrome, and proctocolitis discussed in Chapter 4. Several of the disorders in which the foods causing a problem are only sometimes associated with a positive test for IgE antibody include atopic dermatitis and the allergic eosinophilic gastrointestinal disorders.

For these various illnesses, the search for tests to identify triggering foods is under way and discussed in detail in Chapter 30. A test that is further along in study is the atopy patch test. The atopy patch test requires that the food be placed on the skin for twenty-four to forty-eight hours. Usually the food is prepared as a slurry or porridge and placed under a small metal cap taped to the skin. In some cases, the food has been mixed in a gelatinous substance, which will also hold it onto the skin. The food is removed after a day or two, and the area where the food had contact is examined over the next two or three days for rash. This type of reaction is reminiscent of what happens with poison ivy. Poison ivy and various chemicals and metals that contact the skin can, in some persons, interact with the skin proteins and cause a slow inflammatory reaction, a type of allergy called *contact dermatitis.* Individuals who are sensitive to items in this fashion will not have an immediate response to a substance on the skin but will develop an itchy, red, scaly patch over the days following an exposure. Allergists and dermatologists typically have performed such tests for chemicals used in cosmetics or metals such as nickel found in some jewelry.

Studies performed primarily in Europe have shown that in children who have atopic dermatitis, a positive patch-test reaction to a particular food is likely to be associated with having a delayed skin rash from the food. This is different than having a positive prick skin test or serum IgE test to a food where the reaction tends to be more immediate, with flaring of atopic dermatitis minutes or hours after the ingestion of the food. However, the studies on patch testing have shown many of the same limitations that are seen with the typical allergy skin tests or blood tests for IgE to foods; that is, some individuals' tests are positive, but they have no problem with the food, and some individuals' tests are negative, but they continue to have problems with the food, as demonstrated by oral food challenges. The variations in responses could be attributed to different ways of performing the patch testing and different ways of interpreting the results of the patch tests. Numerous investigations of these patch tests used to diagnose the role of foods in atopic dermatitis and allergic gastrointestinal diseases are ongoing. At this time, the tests are not widely used because their interpretation is not well explored. Additional tests under investigation are discussed in Chapter 30.

Unproven Methods for Diagnosing Food Allergies

I met 11-month-old Andrew to evaluate the possible role of food allergies in his severe atopic dermatitis. I had explained to Andrew's parents the importance of a skin-care regimen to help his skin as much as possible. We were also going to be performing some allergy tests to get a better idea of what foods and environmental allergens were a problem for him. The family had already altered his diet, and I had reviewed the problems that led them to remove certain foods. Following a thorough discussion, I had narrowed the number of possible problem foods to seven or eight that I wanted to evaluate. I explained to Andrew's parents that I would be performing allergy prick skin tests and also serum tests for IgE antibodies for the several foods that might be problematic. I explained limitations of the tests I would perform. Sometimes tests were positive but the food could be tolerated, and sometimes tests were negative for a problematic food. I explained how I would use Andrew's medical history along with my knowledge about Andrew's illness and the test results to identify possible food allergens, but we would still need to perform elimination diets and oral food challenges to reach a diagnosis.

Andrew's family was receptive to the information, but they told me that he had already been evaluated for food allergies. Andrew's mother had undergone muscle-strength testing. She was instructed to hold Andrew and also to hold a jar of Andrew's infant baby food or formula. If the food she was holding was a problem for Andrew, her strength was lessened, but if she was holding a food that Andrew would tolerate, her strength remained. In this way, several foods were determined to be safe for Andrew, and several foods were determined to be problematic.

In listening to this explanation, I could see how straightforward this muscle-strength testing procedure had been. Unlike my complex explanation of allergy test that could be positive and meaningless or even negative and still meaningless, and the need for trial-and-error experimentation with Andrew's diet, the muscle-strength testing procedure seemed definitive, straightforward, and intuitive. As a physician and scientist, even without performing studies to determine whether these muscle-strength testing procedures were valid, I could see no rational explanation why holding your child and a food in a jar would affect your muscle strength and reflect an allergic reaction. Still the logic made sense: something good for you makes you strong and something bad for you makes you weak.

A variety of diagnostic methods have been used by various practitioners over the years but are considered to be "unproved and experimental" by professional allergy organizations, such as the American Academy of Allergy, Asthma and Immunology. Typically, a procedure is considered unproved and experimental when there are no definitive tests to support whether the procedure is helpful in diagnosing a food allergy. Some approaches have not been studied with regard to their effectiveness, and others have been studied but proved ineffective.

Another form of diagnosis, which has also extended into treatment, is *provocation-neutralization therapy.* In this procedure, various extracts of foods are either injected or placed under the tongue, and the person being tested is evaluated for symptoms. Often, the symptoms are subjective, such as weakness or discomfort. Gradually increasing amounts of the food being tested are given to provoke symptoms and then a neutralizing dose is given that abolishes the symptoms. In studies where practitioners used blinded materials with extracts that did or did not (a placebo) contain the foods being tested, the same outcomes were observed. This result indicates that there is a strong suggestive component to this type of procedure.

Various practitioners have used other procedures to diagnose food allergies. Analyzing hair samples, observing blood samples under a microscope as food is added to see whether the food disturbs the cells, and testing electrical resistance through the skin are examples of unproven tests. The pulse test evaluated the subject's pulse rate and strength as various foods were given or discussed. Most of these procedures have fallen from favor because they have not been proved to diagnose food allergy.

Ania is a 9-year-old who had been experiencing headaches and behavioral issues that her family had associated with possible food allergies. The family had read about a test where a blood sample could be sent to a laboratory and analyzed for nearly one hundred foods using a procedure that detected both IgE and IgG antibodies. IgG antibodies are a type of protein formed by the immune system. These antibodies are used to attack germs, such as ones that may travel in the bloodstream. Ania's pediatrician sent a blood sample, and the family received information that showed the test results and suggested treatment diets. Ania had tested positive for many foods that were common in her diet, including typical allergens such as milk, eggs, wheat, and soy. She also tested positive for certain fruits, vegetables, and meats. Her tests were positive for IgG antibodies to these foods. The family had undertaken a variety of manipulations of the diet, and they were not sure whether her symptoms had truly improved.

I explained to Ania's family that a normal immune system produces IgG to various foods in the diet. It is, therefore, possible to detect various degrees of this response in individuals with no food allergies. A few studies have looked at the IgG response to particular food proteins in relationship to symptoms, usually intestinal symptoms. Some of these studies have shown a slight elevation of IgG responses to specific foods when gastrointestinal symptoms are active and a decrease when the gastrointestinal symptoms are inactive. Because the production of IgG is a normal response to the ingestion of foods, one possible explanation for this finding is that an illness in the intestines may allow ingested foods to gain access into the bloodstream more easily, triggering a stronger IgG response. That is, the IgG response may be a reflection of the illness rather than a cause of the illness. Even as a reflection of the illness, not many studies have definitively associated commercial tests of IgG with outcomes in regard to food-specific therapies.

Several studies in adults address IgG testing for medical complaints. A practitioner evaluated the complaints, performed IgG testing, and had the patients remove the IgG-positive foods from their diet. The practitioner then followed up with the patients to see how they were doing. They generally reported an improvement in their symptoms. Unfortunately, this type of study was prone to bias because the complaints varied widely from problems such as weakness to headaches and intestinal symptoms, and the persons affected knew they were changing their own diet. Therefore, it is easy to imagine that they may have had expectations of an improvement. This type of study is not adequate to prove that the test is helpful. Testing for food-specific IgG antibodies in regard to specific food allergies has been considered unproved and experimental by the American Academy of Allergy, Asthma and Immunology, and other experts in professional organizations. While additional research studies continue, this type of testing for allergic responses cannot be recommended at this time.

Ania's specific symptoms were not usually associated with an immune response to foods, and I did not feel that any type of immune system testing would be relevant. We discussed dietary elimination and oral food challenge and whether the family had strong feelings that her symptoms were associated with the foods. I also explained that some food components found in fermented foods and hard cheeses could be associated with triggering headaches in persons with migraines.

A medical history and food-specific IgE antibody tests may not definitively diagnose food allergies. This usually means that to confirm a diagnosis, an oral food challenge is necessary, sometimes with an elimination diet if symptoms are chronic. The IgE antibody tests are limited because they miss the role of foods in certain disorders; therefore, additional tests are under study. The atopy patch test may possibly identify foods that may trigger these non-IgE-mediated responses, but research is needed before the test can be widely recommended. Unfortunately, over the years, many procedures touted for diagnosing food allergies have been ineffective. Some procedures considered unproven or experimental are still in use. When my patients ask whether they should undergo these procedures, I explain the current limitation in our knowledge and the possible role of subjective expectations that may appear to make some of these procedures useful. I would not absolutely prevent my patients from exploring some of these alternative modalities of diagnosis if they are strongly compelled to do so, but I do warn them that the procedures have not been proved and that altering the diet for unproven reasons can be risky. These risks can include nutritional deficits from avoiding an array of foods or allergic reactions from foods to which a child is actually allergic.

13 ~ Putting It All Together

It is not your responsibility to diagnose your own child's food allergies. However, understanding how a doctor performs and interprets a food allergy evaluation can be helpful in many ways. Understanding some of the concepts required for diagnosing a food allergy will empower you to help your doctor make the right diagnosis in your own child. As you have learned, a diagnosis requires a careful and detailed medical history and physical examination, which will lead your doctor to certain suspicions and expectations about what may be causing your child's problems. With a thorough history, your doctor can consider what foods may be problematic. These decisions would result in a selection of tests to be undertaken. Once the tests are performed, it is necessary to understand how they are interpreted and what their limitations may be. Ultimately, putting together many facets of the evaluation can result in an appropriate final diagnosis, and an effective management plan to make life safer for your child and to improve any symptoms. In this chapter, we will use what we have learned to arrive at a diagnosis in three common situations: a child who has experienced anaphylaxis to an unknown trigger, a child who is experiencing chronic symptoms that could be attributed to food allergies and possibly multiple food allergies, and a child who has had symptoms not usually associated with food allergy.

Evaluation of a Sudden Allergic Reaction

Nicole is a 2-year-old with who has a history of asthma. She had eaten a bakery cookie, and two minutes later, her mouth was itchy. Five minutes later, she had hives. Within ten minutes, her lips had swollen and her voice was hoarse. Her mother called the pediatrician who reviewed these symptoms and was certain that the cookie had caused an allergic reaction. Nicole was treated in the emergency room to control her symptoms, and she was sent home with instructions to follow up with her pediatrician. Several days later, Nicole met with her pediatrician who asked about the contents of the cookie. The family contacted the bakery and found out Nicole had eaten an almond cookie made with egg, wheat, and sugar. Nicole had been eating egg and wheat in her diet, but she had never tried nuts. At this point, almond was suspected as the likely cause of the reaction because it was a new food for Nicole and nuts are common allergens. The pediatrician performed blood tests for food allergies and, a few days later, called the family to tell them that the following results had been obtained: egg class 2, wheat class 4, almond class 0, and peanut class 2.

Let us consider what these tests results may mean. The test with the highest value was wheat. However, you will recall that a positive test does not necessarily mean that the person will have a problem ingesting the food. Even though this was the highest test result of the four items tested, and was an ingredient of the cookie, having this test result does not necessarily mean that Nicole was wheat-allergic. In fact, Nicole had been eating wheat up until the time of her reaction and had continued to eat wheat after the reaction with no problems. One could conclude that there was no reason to test for wheat allergy in the first place.

The next highest value was for egg, which is a common food allergen. Although egg was an ingredient in the cookie, it is another food that Nicole eats without a problem, just like wheat. One could again argue that there was not a strong reason to test for egg allergy.

The test for peanut was also positive. The pediatrician had not really discussed whether Nicole ate peanuts or peanut products. In fact, she had. Nicole had not stopped eating peanuts even after this reaction had occurred, and so the positive test to peanut, although it could be associated with allergic reactions in some children, apparently did not indicate a problem for Nicole.

The surprise on these tests was the almond result. One might have expected almond to be positive because we had learned that Nicole did not regularly eat nuts, a common allergen. Almond, although a food related to rock fruits like apples, could potentially cause a significant allergic reaction, and it was a relatively new food for Nicole. When evaluating a sudden allergic reaction to foods, it is usually safe to assume that it is more likely that a reaction occurred to a food that is not a common, previously tolerated part of the diet, compared with a food that is already tolerated in the diet. One could have argued that the only test needed to be done was for almond because Nicole was already eating eggs, wheat, and peanuts. However, the negative almond test raised additional questions.

Nicole's parents brought her and her blood test to my office. They were concerned about the positive tests. But I was concerned about the negative test to almond. It seemed quite likely that almond would have been a problem. Because the blood test for allergy is somewhat less sensitive than a skin test for allergy, I was inclined to do a prick skin test for almond. However, another important point from the history was that this was a bakery cookie. I called the bakery and discovered that the bakery also uses walnuts, cashews, and pecans in many of their products. They admitted that their almond cookies could contain any of the other tree nuts. Nicole's family confirmed that Nicole had never knowingly eaten these other nuts. The prick skin test I performed for almond was negative; however, the prick skin tests for walnuts, cashews, and pecan were strongly positive. Nicole was diagnosed with a tree nut allergy.

Nicole was instructed to avoid any tree nuts and tree nut products, and we spent time reviewing how the family would help her avoid these particular foods. Nicole did not need to avoid peanuts, which she was enjoying, when they were in a form uncontaminated by tree nuts. I also reviewed with the family a plan for emergency treatment in the event that she was to ingest one of these nuts accidentally. If a sudden allergic reaction occurs, a proper diagnosis requires one to consider all the circumstances of the reaction, including possible triggers, foods in the current diet, and foods likely to cause reactions in most people.

Evaluation of a Food Allergy for a Chronic Disease

Jerry is a 2-year-old with severe atopic dermatitis. His family had indicated that he had sudden reactions with hives and vomiting whenever he had eaten eggs or milk. The family was now strictly avoiding all egg and milk products in his foods. However, they also associated an increase in his skin rash to soy, wheat, apple, oat, rice, corn, barley, banana, pear, sweet potato, melon, white potato, pea, and carrot. His current diet consisted of a special hypoallergenic formula and also plum, peach, chicken, beef, spinach, broccoli, and spelt. I reviewed with Jerry's family in great detail the potential environmental exposures that could be triggering his eczema and explained that there are many triggers for atopic dermatitis beyond food allergies. We discussed ways to minimize exposures to environmental allergens to which he might be reactive, and we also discussed a detailed skin-care regimen to try to improve his skin. He came back to see me a few weeks later and still had a significant rash. He was continuing to require large amounts of medications to treat the rash and was uncomfortable.

We chose to undertake both skin and blood testing to determine further what foods might be causing his symptoms. Of course, I wanted to consider the foods that he had already clearly reacted to with sudden allergic symptoms and the foods the family believed to be a trigger for his rash. But most important, I wanted to evaluate the foods that he was currently eating because if any foods were responsible for his rashes, they would be among the ones that he was currently eating. A diet record disclosed the foods in his diet. The following chart shows the size (diameter) of Jerry's skin tests in millimeters (mm) and also the result of his blood tests for IgE to particular foods, measured in units of kIU/L. Test reports include the use of symbols: "<" means less than, and ">" means greater than. The results are organized according to what he was eating or not eating and what was suspected to cause a problem.

	Skin test (in mm)	*Blood IgE result (in U/L)*
Eating		
Plum	3	0.5
Peach	2	0.7
Chicken	4	2.3
Beef	5	44.0
Spelt	Not done	Not done
Suspected to cause a reaction		
Soy	3	8.0
Wheat	7	>100
Apple	3	<0.35
Rice	3	2.0
Pea	3	4.2
Corn	2	3.1
Barley	0	<0.35
Banana	0	1.1
Sweet potato	0	<0.35
Sudden reaction		
Milk	8	>100
Egg	4	7.2
Never eaten		
Peanut	Not done	67.0
Codfish	Not done	47.0

If we ignored our general knowledge about foods that typically cause problems for children with atopic dermatitis, and if we did not consider Jerry's specific history, the test results would be a confusing jumble of numbers. However, the results make sense and add important insight when one considers Jerry's history and information about the foods involved. With regard to the foods he was currently eating, plum, peach, and chicken are not very common foods to cause allergic reactions in individuals with atopic dermatitis. Indeed, his test results to these foods were not particularly strongly positive. I could be somewhat suspicious of chicken, but even that result was not very strong, and it would not be at the top of my list of foods contributing to Jerry's dermatitis.

However, Jerry's tests to beef were very strongly positive. We knew that Jerry has severe milk allergy and that about 10 percent of children with significant milk allergy will react to beef, especially if it is not well cooked. Beef was a common component of Jerry's diet, and on the basis of test results and the knowledge about the role of beef and its relationship to milk, this would be a food I would want Jerry to now avoid.

I did not have a test for spelt, but spelt is a food that is highly related to wheat. The family had already suspected that wheat was a problem, and Jerry had a large skin test and very strong blood test to wheat, indicating a high chance that wheat was a problem food for Jerry. Because of the history of possible wheat allergy and the strong positive tests to wheat, I concluded that spelt might also be an allergen for Jerry. Therefore, to summarize, among the foods that Jerry was eating, beef and spelt should be off-limits.

Jerry's family compiled a list of foods they suspected were problematic. Many of these foods do not usually cause a problem for children with atopic dermatitis. His tests for soy were actually quite low. Among children who have been evaluated for soy allergy, comparing whether they truly react when they undergo a physician-supervised oral food challenge to soy compared with their test results, his results were in a range where most children tolerate soy, and I felt that he could actually include soy in his diet. Jerry was scheduled to eat soy under my supervision as an oral food challenge. He never had a sudden reaction to apple, rice, pea, corn, barley, banana, or sweet potato and had eaten them at various times in his life. His family was not sure these foods had caused problems for him except for possible flares of his atopic dermatitis. After discussing how atopic dermatitis naturally increases and decreases, and after seeing these low values to these suspected foods, it seemed unlikely that any of them were a problem for him.

We were not going to have Jerry ingest milk or egg because these had caused sudden allergic reactions for him before. Indeed, his test results to these two foods documented a high likelihood of current allergy. Children with tests such as these would be expected to have a greater than 95 percent risk to have reactions to milk or egg, although the severity of the reaction is not predictable by these results. I also tested two highly allergenic foods that Jerry had not yet ingested. Unfortunately, both the tests for peanut and codfish were in ranges where reactions are expected. I reviewed with Jerry's family that he should not be exposed to these foods. Soy could be added back to his diet under my supervision as an oral food challenge. We confirmed that most foods that were a part of his diet were likely to be safe, but spelt and beef would be removed.

The family had considered that melon was a problem. This was one food that I do not have a reliable test for because proteins in melon change when it is left to stand, say, in a bottle waiting for allergy skin testing. I would need the family to bring in fresh melon so I could perform a skin test with the fresh, raw juice. However, melon also has proteins that are very similar to proteins in ragweed pollen. An individual with ragweed allergy may react to melon because of the similar proteins. Further evaluation disclosed that Jerry was allergic to ragweed, which might explain why his rash flared during ragweed season and made me suspect a reaction to melon. I performed a skin test with the fresh melon juice his family brought in, and he had a strong positive skin test. The family's instincts about the melon were right.

I explained to Jerry's family the various issues in avoiding foods to which he was allergic, and we reviewed an emergency care plan for treatment of anaphylaxis. We discussed the avoidance of the foods we identified and undertook oral challenges to expand his diet. Jerry did well; the rash diminished, his sleep improved, and he required fewer medications.

Evaluation of a Complaint That Is Not Likely to Be a Food Allergy

Maya is a 4-year-old whose parents brought her to see me because of headaches. Maya would develop sudden headaches and scream in discomfort. She would run to either a couch, pillow, or chair and press her head deeply into the cushions. She would do this for ten to twenty minutes after eating certain foods. She would tell her parents that she had a headache and would cry, and they would give her headache medication for these episodes. The family came to see me because they were concerned that certain foods were triggering these headaches.

Headaches are not a common symptom of food allergy. In some individuals, migraine headaches are triggered by certain food components found, for example, in fermented foods, but Maya's pattern of headaches seemed unusual because the headaches came on so suddenly, were severe, and did not last very long, unlike migraine headaches. After a few more questions, it was clear that Maya had no family history of migraine headaches, but I also learned that Maya had experienced some allergic problems, particularly hay fever and mild asthma. Family history did indicate allergies.

I asked the family to describe the particular foods that had caused her headaches. Apples, peaches, and hazelnuts seemed to cause her headaches. The headaches always came on within minutes of ingesting these foods. I also learned that she was able to tolerate apple juice or applesauce with no problem, and similarly she had eaten peach pie and canned peaches without a problem. The fresh, or raw, form of apple and peach seemed to cause these headaches. I suspected that Maya was having a food-allergic reaction. By gathering more information, I learned that Maya began having these episodes when she was about 2½-years-old. Around that time, her mother noticed that with these particular foods, she would behave in the manner described, by pressing her face into the furniture and crying. Her mother would say to her, "Do you have a headache? Do you have a headache?" Maya quickly learned to use the word "headache" whenever she experienced these episodes. I wondered, then, whether these episodes were ever headaches. Because Maya had a history of hay fever and reacted to foods that contain proteins related to birch pollen, I wondered whether she had oral allergy syndrome. In fact, her family also reported that she made clucking noises and would put her fingers in her ears during these episodes, which are signs of trying to scratch an itchy throat. I explained to the family about pollen-food-related syndrome, or oral allergy syndrome. This is a food allergy in which an individual becomes allergic to pollen and then experiences symptoms from certain foods that have similar proteins. Heat destroys the protein, which explained why she could tolerate apple juice, applesauce, and canned peaches and peach pie but not the raw fruit.

Maya was probably experiencing an itchy mouth accompanied by an itchy sensation inside the ears or on her forehead. She was rubbing her head and squirming herself into the couch or chair to scratch her itch. She was not really experiencing a headache but had learned through her mother's prompting from an early age that these types of symptoms might be called "headache." We skin tested Maya, and she was indeed positive to birch pollen and also to juices from fresh apple and peach, but she was negative to our commercial extracts of peach and apple, which do not contain the same protein as the raw versions. Maya would continue to avoid the several foods that were birch pollen related, but she would continue to eat several other types of foods that were related to birch pollen that had never caused a problem for her. We discussed that this is generally a mild type of allergy, but there was a small chance that more significant symptoms could occur, and we discussed emergency preparedness in case that were to happen.

For evaluating an anaphylactic reaction, or for the possibility of food allergy triggering a chronic disease, or even when there is an unusual situation that may not typically be associated with a food allergy, it is important to put together the details of the history and also to apply a broad knowledge of the features of food allergic diseases and the foods that can cause them. Testing can then be decided on and interpreted in the context of all of these features to arrive at the most appropriate diagnosis. It is also important, of course, to keep an open mind to alternative possibilities such as disorders that can cause similar medical problems but are not food allergies or the possibility of unusual symptoms that are actually caused by a food allergy.

PART 3

TREATING AN ALLERGIC REACTION

When your child has been diagnosed with a potentially life-threatening food allergy, your doctor will prescribe medications to use in the event of an allergic reaction. Epinephrine is the primary medication used to reverse the most severe symptoms of an allergic or anaphylactic reaction. Other medications may be used outside of the hospital setting, and additional medications and treatments are available to your child in an emergency department should the reaction require advanced therapies. In Chapter 2, I described the features of an anaphylactic reaction and discussed what may differentiate an anaphylactic reaction from a milder allergic reaction. When a reaction is, or is likely to become, anaphylaxis, epinephrine must be injected promptly. In Part 3, I discuss various features of the medications used to treat anaphylactic and allergic reactions to foods. You will also see how these medications are just one part of a larger emergency care plan used to keep your child safe.

In a study regarding the use of emergency medications for anaphylaxis, a family's comfort with using emergency medications was associated with several factors, including previous experience with the medication and understanding how to use medications. But the factor that was most strongly associated with appropriate use of emergency medications was the feeling of empowerment. Empow-

erment in regard to medical emergencies means that you feel you can handle a crisis calmly, confidently, decisively, accurately, and quickly. Achieving this type of comfort requires understanding the use and actions of the medications for treating an allergic reaction and having an organized plan in place should your child need to be treated.

14 ~ Epinephrine

Epinephrine, which is sometimes referred to as *adrenaline,* is a medication that reverses all of the more dangerous symptoms of a severe allergic reaction. Epinephrine makes the heart beat stronger and faster to improve blood circulation. It tightens floppy blood vessels, allowing these blood vessels to channel blood more efficiently to all of the vital organs. Epinephrine relaxes twitchy breathing tubes to reverse the symptoms of asthma. It reduces the leakiness of blood vessels so that there is less swelling. It may also reduce some of the itching and hives and may also relieve some of the gastrointestinal symptoms that occur during anaphylaxis. Your or your child's body naturally produces epinephrine or adrenaline during what is called the "fight-or-flight" response. The fight-or-flight response refers to a situation where a person is faced with fear or danger, and the adrenal gland in the body pumps out adrenaline that results in a burst of increased energy, heart racing, and physical strength to either fight a danger or to run away from one. In the face of an anaphylactic allergic reaction, an injection of epinephrine provides the means to reverse the life-threatening symptoms of anaphylaxis, giving your child time to get to an emergency room for additional therapies if they are needed.

It is dramatic to consider injecting a medication into your own child or having your child self-inject. However, epinephrine was used to treat asthma attacks before asthma inhalers were formulated. For example, an individual having breathing difficulties from asthma would see her doctor. The physician would inject a dose of epinephrine and have the person rest for a while as the symptoms of asthma dissipated. Perhaps an individual would feel the asthma symptoms coming on a while later. In that case, they would get additional injections of epinephrine. Epinephrine is still used to treat severe asthma attacks. However, the inhaled medications are quite effective for asthma and have essentially replaced the use of epinephrine in most situations.

Most of epinephrine's side effects are expected and based on the action of the drug. That is, the heart may race and the person may feel jittery as could occur, for example, after drinking a large amount of a caffeinated beverage such as coffee. An individual may appear pale or, in some cases, a bit flushed. Familiarity with the effects of epinephrine is key because, unfortunately, some symptoms resemble anaphylactic symptoms. For example, epinephrine may cause heart racing or a feeling of apprehension, sweating, or anxiety. Epinephrine may also cause a headache and weakness. These side effects are generally short-lived, occurring just for a number of minutes after the treatment. More significant symptoms from the epinephrine can occur, but these are rare, except for individuals who have heart disease or are elderly. Because epinephrine makes the heart beat fast, if an individual has heart disease that can be worsened by a fast heart rate, the epinephrine may pose this additional concern. You should discuss these issues with your doctor if your child has any heart disease or other medical problems. Epinephrine can also interact with certain medications such as ones used to treat depression, blood pressure, or heart problems. However, in an otherwise healthy child, usual doses of epinephrine administered for anaphylaxis would not be expected to cause severe problems. In fact, even for individuals who have heart problems and are at risk of having worse side effects from epinephrine because of an increased heart rate, the primary instructions remain: to use epinephrine to treat anaphylaxis despite any increased risk.

I generally prescribe self-injectable epinephrine for a child who has experienced an anaphylactic reaction or is at increased risk to experience one. An allergist or pediatrician may consider many factors in deciding who should be prescribed self-injectable epinephrine.

Some of the difficult decisions that have to be made in deciding whether to prescribe self-injectable epinephrine came up when I saw Cassy, an 11-month-old girl who had experienced hives and coughing after she was fed eggs for the first time. It was not clear that Cassy had a severe allergic reaction because her primary symptom after eating the eggs was hives and a mild cough. Egg allergy is usually not considered a severe allergy, and some pediatricians or allergists would probably not prescribe self-injectable epinephrine. However, in my discussion with Cassy's family, circumstances indicated that Cassy had a modest risk of severe reactions to foods in the future. Although Cassy was 11 months old, she seemed prone to wheezing and now had evidence of a food allergy. It was possible that she would continue to have problems with wheezing and develop additional food allergies. It was a good decision to have the family prepared by having self-injectable epinephrine.

Prescribing self-injectable epinephrine is a big decision; it can have a very strong effect on how a family views a child. For example, the prescription may worry a family, making them think of their child as sickly or vulnerable. I explained to Cassy's family that she was not at a high risk of a fatal reaction and that the self-injectable epinephrine would be her life insurance policy. Chances were good that she would not need it, but I felt secure knowing she would have it if the need arose. Still, plenty of issues remained for the family to discuss.

The first issue was about prescribing the correct dose of self-injectable epinephrine. In the United States and in other countries where self-injector devices are available, they have been developed with two doses that are not adjustable. A device formulated for children contains an amount of 0.15 milligrams of epinephrine, and a device formulated for older children or adults contains 0.30 milligram of epinephrine. You may see the word "milligram" abbreviated as "mg" in the packaging, and this abbreviation will be used in the remainder of this book. Manufacturers generally recommend using the lower dose for children weighing 33 pounds to 66 pounds and the larger dose for those weighing over 66 pounds. However, the manufacturers acknowledge that a doctor may prescribe one of these devices for an individual outside of the recommended weight ranges when considering issues specific to that particular child.

Guidelines have suggested that the 0.15 mg dose is just right for someone who weighs 33 pounds (also known in the metric system as 15 kilograms, or kg) and the 0.30 mg dose is just right for someone who weighs 66 pounds (or 30 kg). With only two doses to choose from, your doctor may determine that it would be better to provide a higher dose to a child who weighs closer to, but less than, 66 pounds. Many allergists will switch children to the 0.30 mg dose when they are about 55 pounds. The doctor may switch them at an even lower weight if they feel that a child is at a particularly high risk of a severe reaction, or they may wait and switch to the higher dose at a higher weight if they feel that the risk of a severe reaction is low.

For Cassy, the problem of selecting an appropriate dose was in the other direction because she only weighed 20 pounds, well below the 33-pound weight suggested for the 0.15 mg preloaded epinephrine injector. The only way to provide Cassy with the exact recommended amount of epinephrine would be to draw it up from a vial into a syringe. There is a possibility that premeasured self-injection devices formulated for infants will eventually be available, but this was not an option at the time I was treating Cassy. I explained to Cassy's family that to give just the right dose for her size, they would need to open a glass vial, insert a needle into the vial, pull back a small amount using small gradations shown on a syringe, remove an air bubble from the syringe, and then inject the medication. Cassy's family was concerned about administering the correct dosage in this manner while she was having a severe allergic reaction. Studies looked at a family's ability to prepare an injection of epinephrine using a vial and syringe; they often made significant dosing errors. Having discussed this, we felt that the safety of using the self-injector dose was a better decision for Cassy than using the glass ampule and syringe. In deciding on the correct dose and method of giving self-injectable epinephrine for your child, a variety of circumstances should be discussed with your physician to find what is best for you and your child.

In the United States, two brands of self-injector devices are available: the EpiPen, which contains 0.30 mg epinephrine, and EpiPen Jr., with a 0.15-mg dose of epinephrine. Another brand is called the Twinject, which is also available in 0.30-mg and 0.15-mg doses. Both of these devices are autoinjectors. The EpiPen provides a single dose per injector unit. The Twinject unit, in a single unit, provides the first dose as a spring-loaded autoinjector, and the second dose is accessed by opening the injector and removing a syringe preloaded with the second dose of epinephrine. For the EpiPen/EpiPen Jr., if a second dose is needed, a second self-injector unit is used. In Part 9, you will find step-by-step instructions for both of these units as part of the Food Allergy Action Plan. In addition, the manufacturers provide Web sites that show videos on the use of these treatments. The decision about which of these units, or units that may be manufactured in the future, is best for you and your child should be discussed with your allergist or pediatrician.

I explained to Cassy's family that whichever unit we decided to prescribe, it was important that they reviewed how the injector works. I and other researchers have performed studies where we have quizzed families on how to use the self-injector. Many families make errors trying to demonstrate correct use. These units come with trainer devices and detailed instructions that must be reviewed. I suggest monthly practices with the trainer devices. You may want to assign yourself a convenient reminder, such as when you pay a monthly bill, to review how the self-injector works.

It is important to properly store the unit and ensure it has not expired. These units should not be refrigerated or exposed to extremes of temperature. This does not mean that they cannot withstand short periods at temperatures outside of room temperature, but they should not be frozen and they should not have prolonged exposure to heat or extremes of temperature. For example, storing them in a glove compartment would not be a good idea because they may get overheated or frozen. Carrying a unit in a purse or a carrying case are safe ways to maintain the proper temperature, or storing it in a cooler may be helpful, at least for short periods of time.

The medication can be seen through a small window on the device. Discolored medication may indicate that it is losing potency. Both manufacturers provide a means to receive reminders when the prescription needs to be renewed. If you are ever faced with an emergency situation where you have not renewed your self-injector but need it, most authorities, including myself, recommend giving the medication if needed rather than giving no medication and delaying treatment. Even if the medication has expired or become discolored, some active medication may remain; it may be worth using this rather than doing nothing. These medications are preserved with sulfite, but it is recommended to use them even if you suspect or have sulfite sensitivity.

During the office visit with Cassy's family, I showed them exactly how to use the self-injector and had them demonstrate, with the trainer's help, that they understood how to give it to Cassy. These injectors typically provide a needle that can reach into the muscle of the leg, which is a location where studies have shown that epinephrine is absorbed very well and quickly. Be sure to review with your doctor exactly how to use the self-injector unit. The needle can go through clothing, but I usually suggest pulling up a dress or pulling down pants to avoid a seam, a buckle, or an object in a pocket.

Cassy's family wanted to know how likely it might be that Cassy would need a second dose during a reaction. Unfortunately, few studies evaluate how often a child might need a second dose of self-injectable epinephrine before reaching the hospital after a food-allergic reaction. In one study with children with food allergies, 10 percent of the children who received a dose of epinephrine needed a second dose, though not necessarily before they came to the hospital. In studies of adults and in studies of anaphylaxis from a variety of sources, including to insect stings and to injections to treat pollen allergies, between 1 in 12 to 1 in 3 reactions were treated with a second dose. Therefore, you should have two doses on hand.

How much time may be allowed between administering the first dose and the second? This is a tricky question because one dose is usually all that is required, but the need for a second dose implies that the child did not respond well to that first dose or that symptoms have returned. I explained to Cassy's family that authorities often say that a second dose would be given five to twenty minutes after the first dose if symptoms were not abating. In reality, if symptoms worsened after that first dose, I would not wait more than several minutes before giving the second dose, keeping in mind, though, that some side effects of the injection of epinephrine, such as a bit of change of color of the skin or faster heart rates, might have been an expected result of that first injection. I discussed with Cassy's family a variety of situations and types of symptoms for which they would treat with the self-injectable epinephrine, as indicated in Chapter 2. Their primary concern was what would happen if they gave the epinephrine and Cassy had not actually needed it? What if they panicked and were unsure? I reassured them that giving epinephrine is generally safe, and if they erred on the side of giving it when perhaps it was not necessary, it was highly unlikely that this would cause any problems for Cassy, who is otherwise healthy. In fact, they might have saved her life.

Epinephrine is the primary medication used in the event of an anaphylactic reaction. It should be injected promptly to reverse potentially dangerous symptoms to give your child the needed time to get to an emergency room. Whichever self-injector or injection device you and your doctor decide on, it is important to review how the medication is used and to make sure that your medication has neither expired nor become discolored. Various carrying cases are on the market to protect the devices from extremes of temperature and to improve the ease of carrying them.

15 ~ Antihistamines and Other Therapies

In addition to epinephrine, a number of other therapies may be used to treat your child's allergic reactions and anaphylaxis. In this chapter, we will review the various treatments that are available to you before you arrive at an emergency room and also medications paramedics or physicians in an emergency room setting may administer.

Antihistamines

Histamine is a chemical released from mast cells and basophils that causes many of the symptoms of an allergic reaction. It makes blood vessels floppy and leaky so that swelling occurs, and it triggers nerves that cause itching. An antihistamine blocks the action of histamine. During more severe allergic reactions, large amounts of histamine may be released before you give your child the antihistamine. Therefore, it is not surprising to see the effects of an allergic reaction, such as swelling, continue for a while, even though an antihistamine was given. However, antihistamines are very helpful in suppressing and, to some extent, preventing many of the common symptoms that occur during an allergic reaction. Some antihistamines are available over the counter and others are prescription medications.

Traditionally, diphenhydramine (e.g., Benadryl) has been used to treat allergic reactions to foods. The liquid form is easy to give to children or young adults and would be absorbed more rapidly into the body than the pill form, which first needs to dissolve in the stomach. New formulations of diphenhydramine that melt in the mouth have also become available. You should discuss with your doctor which formulation may best fit your child. Even though a liquid may be used, the medication does not usually take effect immediately. The antihistamine could take thirty to sixty minutes to take effect.

Sleepiness is a side effect of diphenhydramine. However, some children actually experience increased activity after a dose of antihistamine. Antihistamines such as diphenhydramine may impair activities because of the drowsiness. This is usually not an issue for children, but it is more of an issue for adults or for teenagers who drive. Some physicians prescribe nonsedating antihistamines for use in the event of an allergic reaction. For example, a medication called *cetirizine* has an onset of action that may be slightly faster than diphenhydramine and is less sedating. There are several types of sedating and nonsedating antihistamines on the market, and you should discuss these choices with your doctor. Most of the antihistamines have few side effects.

The role of an antihistamine in anaphylaxis is to provide additional relief of symptoms. It should *not* be relied on to improve the life-threatening symptoms of an anaphylactic reaction. However, there are many circumstances where a child may experience mild symptoms of an allergic reaction and an antihistamine can be provided for relief. An antihistamine can be given for any type of allergic reaction, but giving the antihistamine should never delay administration of epinephrine if the epinephrine is needed.

Sidney is a 7-year-old who uses a nonsedating antihistamine each day for her hay fever. Sidney also has a peanut allergy, and her family had several questions about the use of antihistamines during an allergic reaction, considering that she was already taking a daily antihistamine. There is a theoretical concern that if a child is on a chronic antihistamine, the child perhaps may not notice mild initial symptoms from a food allergic reaction that would otherwise alert them that they have ingested the food to which they are allergic. Most experts, including myself, would not deny a child, because of a theoretical concern, a good treatment for a chronic condition such as hay fever that would otherwise disturb them. One could argue that being on a chronic antihistamine may reduce the chance of having allergic symptoms from small exposures, but in that regard, most doctors would not typically prescribe an antihistamine as a preventative for food allergic reactions. For Sidney's emergency plan, we decided to include the treatment of diphenhydramine, in addition to self-injectable epinephrine, in the event of a severe reaction. We decided on diphenhydramine rather than her usually nonsedating antihistamine because other individuals in Sidney's school had also been prescribed the same medication, and it seemed like a good decision for her plan to be similar to the ones used by others in her class.

Sidney's family wondered whether they should alter her emergency plan because she typically received an antihistamine each morning for her hay fever. Should she not receive another dose if she had an allergic reaction at school? An additional amount of antihistamine, even if it were given soon after her morning dose, would not be a problem. It was more important to maintain uniformity of her plan and the additional amount of antihistamine would not be a danger to her. You should discuss these types of issues with your doctor so that a plan is in place ahead of time should an allergic reaction occur while your child is taking antihistamines for other reasons.

Antihistamines are an important additional medication in the treatment of anaphylaxis and are the primary medication for treating mild allergic reactions. They usually do not take effect for 30 to 60 minutes after they are ingested, so improvement may not occur right away. Of course, if symptoms progressed toward an anaphylactic reaction, epinephrine would be the medication needed.

Medications Used for Asthma

Sheila is a 9-year-old with multiple food allergies and asthma. Her asthma care includes the use of an inhaled steroid medication and a rescue inhaler called *albuterol,* which provides relief in the event of coughing, wheezing, or chest tightness. She has also used a pill called an *antileukotriene.* Sheila's mother wondered what she should do about using her asthma medications in the event that Sheila experienced a severe allergic reaction to any of the foods that she tries to avoid. I explained that studies show that individuals with food allergy and asthma are at increased risk of a more severe reaction should they ingest the food to which they are allergic. This is probably because it is more likely that the asthma-prone lungs would be affected during an allergic reaction to food, resulting in severe symptoms. For these reasons, it was important to keep Sheila's asthma under the best control possible.

Several of the medications that Sheila used reduced lung inflammation, a major cause of problems for asthma. These medications included the antileukotriene and the inhaled steroid. Antileukotrienes block one aspect of inflammation and are prescribed for treating both asthma and allergic rhinitis (hay fever) symptoms; in theory, they may also block one of the chemicals produced during an anaphylactic reaction, but this has not been studied. Steroids, either inhaled or oral, quell many of the immune cells that add to lung inflammation that contributes to asthma. Individuals like Sheila who have asthma may be prescribed other medications to reduce lung inflammation. In fact, Sheila had used one such drug, cromolyn, in the past. The various medications that reduce inflammation in lungs help control asthma, but they do not generally work right away and would not be medications to reach for during an asthma "attack."

Next, Sheila's family and I discussed the use of her bronchodilator in the event of an allergic reaction. Bronchodilators work by relaxing the tiny rings of muscle that surround the breathing tubes. The muscles twitch during asthma and squeeze the breathing tubes, making it harder for air to pass, resulting in the wheezing noise. The bronchodilator asthma "rescue" medication works quickly to improve breathing. Sheila typically carried her rescue inhaler with her, and I explained that she should use the inhaler to help relieve breathing problems during a sudden allergic reaction to foods. *However, it was vital that she realize, and that all of her caregivers realize, that albuterol should not substitute for epinephrine.* In fact, giving her epinephrine would also relieve her breathing problems, while also improving her circulation and other symptoms of anaphylaxis.

The albuterol would reach the surface of the lung and improve breathing, but it would not improve all of the different areas of the body that epinephrine could help during an episode of anaphylaxis. For example, the albuterol would not reduce the throat swelling or improve the blood circulation. Thus, the albuterol could and should be used during an allergic reaction if Sheila were experiencing asthma symptoms. However, it should not be relied on as a primary treatment for anaphylaxis. *Deaths from anaphylaxis have been attributed to a victim's reliance on the use of an asthma inhaler instead of an injection of epinephrine.* "Long-acting" bronchodilators, such as salmeterol, should not be used as emergency treatment of an asthma attack or during anaphylaxis; the short-acting bronchodilators, such as albuterol, should be used.

Steroids

An allergic reaction occurs when various chemicals are released by cells of the immune system. Steroid medications, not the kind that build muscles but the kind that reduce inflammation, work by calming down the various immune system cells. Inhaled steroids are used for asthma to reduce inflammation in the lung, and nasal steroids are used in the nose to reduce nasal inflammation when a person has nasal allergies. While these medications are useful for treating chronic illnesses such as hay fever and asthma, they would not be considered emergency medications for treatment of anaphylaxis for several reasons. First, they are only working in a location where they are being sprayed, and second, they take a long time to reduce inflammation.

Steroids can also be given by mouth or injected. When they are given in this way, they travel throughout the body and reduce inflammation virtually everywhere. Still, it takes hours for these treatments to take effect. You would guess that steroids would be helpful in treating an allergic reaction because they would be calming the immune system response throughout the body. When there is a severe allergic reaction, steroids are often given. The theory behind giving the steroids is that they would reduce reactions that may occur after there has been a severe allergic reaction. You may recall that sometimes anaphylaxis will respond to initial treatments, but then a second wave of symptoms, called a *biphasic response,* will sometimes occur. Some individuals continue to have anaphylaxis for many hours or several days. Steroids are often given when there has been a severe allergic reaction, with the hope that they will quell later allergic responses. Steroids would, therefore, not be part of an immediate action plan for treatment of anaphylaxis symptoms, but they are often added for an individual who has had a severe reaction. No studies have been conducted on the effectiveness of providing steroids to individuals experiencing anaphylaxis to determine whether the steroids alter the course of anaphylaxis. If you have sought medical attention, for example, in an emergency room or a doctor's office, and your child has been diagnosed with a severe reaction, your doctor may administer and prescribe these steroids. Some physicians will recommend taking the steroids for a day or two after an allergic reaction has occurred. This judgment will be based on the severity of the reaction.

Advanced Therapies for Anaphylaxis

If you have used epinephrine or if you have considered administering epinephrine and are uncertain about the severity of your child's reaction or whether the symptoms are progressing, I always recommend taking your child to the emergency room. In an emergency room, personnel and equipment are available to evaluate and manage allergic reactions and anaphylaxis. During an anaphylactic reaction, the blood pressure may be low. This is anaphylactic shock. It occurs when the heart is not pumping well and the blood vessels have become floppy. In addition to treatment with epinephrine, intravenous fluids are used to help support blood pressure during severe anaphylaxis. These fluids can be provided in an emergency room or by paramedics during transport to the emergency room. Because lung function and circulation are impaired, providing oxygen is an important additional therapy. Ambulances and emergency rooms are equipped with materials needed to provide additional oxygen to your child should this be required.

Additional medications can be given to help support failing organs during a severe anaphylactic reaction. Advanced treatments are not usually needed, but they are available in most paramedic-equipped ambulances and also in emergency departments. Such medications include intravenous medications that help to support blood pressure and heart function. During anaphylaxis, some experts recommend providing not only typical antihistamines used for allergy but also a type of histamine blocker used to treat acid reflux disease, which may be used in the emergency room. In extreme circumstances, say, if swelling around the windpipe occurs, advanced therapy could include inserting a breathing tube into the windpipe and assisting breathing with a ventilator. Although various advanced therapies are usually not needed in an anaphylactic reaction, it is important to get medical attention where they are available and where doctors can monitor and treat your child accordingly.

Additional Therapies under Investigation

Activated charcoal, which is not like the charcoal used in a barbecue, is a medical treatment used for some types of poisonings. It is either swallowed or inserted through a tube into the stomach and can absorb toxins that were ingested in the event of a poisoning. One study evaluated the ability of activated charcoal to bind up and absorb peanut proteins. The activated charcoal appeared to be helpful in doing this in a test tube. Should activated charcoal be added to the list of treatments used in the event of an allergic reaction outside of a hospital setting? Most experts believe that activated charcoal cannot, at this time, be recommended for routine use for food allergy for several reasons. No studies have been conducted to show whether it is effective for absorbing food allergens in the stomach during an allergic reaction. More important, the treatment does not taste good and can often result in vomiting and would be very difficult to give to a child during an allergic reaction. The activated charcoal would also likely bind and therefore inactivate an antihistamine that was taken. Last, should a reaction become more severe, vomiting is possible, and if a child is having trouble breathing and vomits after having the charcoal, the child could accidentally inhale the charcoal, which can cause lung damage. For all of these reasons, activated charcoal has not been suggested as part of therapy for a food-allergic reaction outside of the hospital setting. In some circumstances, individual physicians may consider using activated charcoal once the child is already under advanced medical care, although studies on its effectiveness in this setting are also lacking.

When an individual experiences a severe anaphylactic reaction and the heart is affected, this is called *anaphylactic shock*. When circulation is very poor, the blood cannot get to vital organs such as the brain and the organs in the chest and abdomen. Symptoms include poor pulse, pale and pasty skin, and altered consciousness. Blood may actually pool in less important places, like the legs. When a person has sudden low blood pressure, it is often recommended that they raise their legs while lying down. This actually allows blood to flow, from gravitational force, from the legs into the main part of the body to the vital organs.

In several adults who experienced severe anaphylaxis, it was observed that when they were lying down, they appeared to be generally stable, but when they were brought up to a sitting or standing position, they suddenly became much sicker and sometimes died. If someone has very low blood pressure, is experiencing anaphylactic shock, and is raised to a sitting or standing position, the blood may pool into the legs and the heart suddenly would have very little blood to pump. This problem may have resulted in fatalities in these several individuals. Whether this is an issue for children is completely unknown. Most children who have an anaphylactic response to food seem to have a more prominent problem with breathing than with circulation. Nonetheless, some experts recommend that if your child is having a severe allergic reaction to food with symptoms of poor circulation, that they be kept in a lying position, legs up, to help circulation and that they be transported to an emergency room for advanced care while they remain in the lying position. However, laying a child down who may be having an asthma response and vomiting could pose its own dangers, such as more trouble breathing or choking. You should discuss these issues with your doctor, but if your child is already having severe anaphylaxis with poor circulation and is in a lying position with legs up, it may be reasonable to continue that position for ambulance transportation until the blood pressure is under better control.

In addition to injected epinephrine for treatment of anaphylaxis, there are a variety of medications such as antihistamines to improve itching and swelling, and asthma medications such as albuterol to relieve breathing problems, that may be used during an allergic reaction. These additional medications can be given promptly to a child who is experiencing an allergic or anaphylactic reaction. It is important to realize that asthma inhalers and antihistamines are additional therapies that are helpful in treating anaphylaxis, but *they do not substitute for epinephrine.* In the event of anaphylaxis, after injecting epinephrine, it is important to seek additional medical care in an emergency room so that medications and treatments such as additional epinephrine, steroids, intravenous fluids, oxygen, or other medications to support breathing and blood pressure are available and can be administered under expert guidance. To treat anaphylaxis, medications are important, but as you will see in Chapter 16, they are only part of an emergency care plan and emergency action plan for treatment of food allergy.

16 ~ Emergency Action Plans for Anaphylaxis

Every child with a potentially life-threatening food allergy should have an emergency care plan in place to prevent and to respond to food-allergic reactions. An emergency care plan is a broad, multifaceted program that includes a variety of components. These components include education of the child and those around the child on how to avoid ingesting the foods the child is allergic to, an understanding of the symptoms that can occur in a food allergic reaction, an appreciation for the medications that are to be used in the event of a reaction and their technique of administration, and a written emergency action plan that describes many of the components of recognizing and treating an allergic reaction, including who should be contacted. The overall plan would include a practice drill to prepare for the possibility of a reaction. A comprehensive emergency care plan would include identifying individuals who are responsible for the child's safety. Many components of this broad emergency care plan are described in other chapters of this book. Here we will focus on components of the plan that involve recognizing the allergic reaction, instituting prompt treatment, and alerting personnel to obtain advanced care.

The Emergency Action Plan

The primary component of an emergency care plan is the written summary outlining key points in treating an allergic or anaphylactic reaction. An example of a written emergency action plan is provided in Part 9, and the most current version of this plan may be obtained through the Food Allergy & Anaphylaxis Network. You should work with your doctor to complete a written food allergy action plan. The plan should identify your child and preferably have a picture of your child on the document. It should identify the foods your child is allergic to. In some cases, I indicate specific foods that are most likely to cause a severe allergic reaction and sometimes differentiate these from additional foods that are less likely to cause a severe reaction but which the child should avoid. The written plan should list potential symptoms and the recommended therapies, which would usually include epinephrine and an antihistamine, depending on the particular symptoms. Because many varieties of written emergency action plans exist, you should discuss with your doctor the best summary form for your child. Many of the examples of anaphylaxis given in Chapter 2 indicate that responses to allergic reactions depend on the symptoms, the food involved, features of past reactions, and the qualifications of the person evaluating your child. Depending on the particular circumstances, these decisions may be reflected in the written action plans. The action plan should specify when to call 911 to summon an ambulance. Contact numbers for parents, guardians, and the child's physicians should be listed.

Families sometimes create individualized emergency action plans tailored to their child's particular circumstances. However, I have also seen emergency care forms that go on for many pages and would be very difficult to use in the event of an emergency. I am not in favor of these. Have your doctor review the written emergency action plan before you submit it to schools, camps, or other caregivers. Forms may need to be modified, depending on the qualifications of individuals caring for your child. For example, the form may give a school nurse leeway to make decisions when to inject epinephrine because the school nurse is a health care professional who is expected to be able to discern symptoms and the need for treatment. In contrast, a plan may suggest injection of epinephrine more liberally if the caregiver is not a health care professional.

Trevor, a 7-year-old with milk, egg, and peanut allergies, had tasted his friend's cookie at school during lunch and experienced an itchy mouth and face. He had an emergency action plan in place. The school nurse was away. The principal was also designated to evaluate a child with an allergic reaction in the nurse's absence. The principal observed that Trevor was coughing and had hives. The principal called Trevor's mother at home. There was no answer, so he left a message there explaining Trevor's allergic reaction. The principal reached Trevor's mother on her cell phone and explained Trevor's condition. Because of a bad connection, the call was cut short. By the time the principal reached Trevor's mother again, she was panic-stricken and urged the principal to follow the emergency action plan. In fact, the principal had the emergency action plan in front of him; it clearly indicated that in the event Trevor likely ate unsafe food and developed a reaction with breathing or respiratory symptoms, epinephrine should be injected. The principal injected the epinephrine, which he had been trained to do, and Trevor felt better. The principal then called 911, and Trevor was taken by ambulance to the emergency room, where his mother met him. He required no further treatment and improved.

The potentially dangerous error that occurred was that the principal delayed giving the medication while he tried to contact the family, rather than following the emergency action plan, which instructed the caregiver to provide medication to Trevor, if warranted, then call an ambulance, and, finally, notify the family. The action plan was fine, but Trevor's caregivers had not reviewed it beforehand.

Trevor did not suffer any severe consequences as a result of the principal's failure to carry out the emergency action plan. The principal was well trained in giving the medication and in recognizing an allergic reaction, but he was not well informed about the sequence of events, which is why practice runs make sense. Each individual involved in the care of your child should review and practice the sequence of events that would be taken in the event of a reaction. As you will see in future chapters, this plan includes many individuals who care for your child and must understand food allergic reactions and their treatment. Of course, your child must be included in understanding the plan. Trevor notified an adult that he was having a problem, even though he might have been shy, embarrassed, or worried considering he had intentionally tasted someone else's cookie. Everyone knew to take Trevor to the school nurse or the principal. Everyone knew where the medications were kept and that an emergency action plan should be followed; however, the error regarding who to contact first could have been avoided had the plan been carefully reviewed.

Medical Identification Jewelry

Three-year-old Toni had been diagnosed with peanut and tree nut allergies and was strictly avoiding these foods. Her mother cared for her at home, and she went to a playgroup three times a week for half a day, during which time she played while her mother supervised. On occasion, a friend supervised Toni in the playgroup. That friend also knew about Toni's food allergies and how to administer her medications. The family wanted to know whether they should obtain medical identification (or alert) jewelry for Toni.

I strongly believe in medical identification jewelry for children with potentially life-threatening food allergies. Several organizations (see Part 9, Keeping Current) provide these bracelets or medallions that carry information about food allergies and anaphylaxis. The information can also be linked with more specific medical details available by accessing a Web site or calling, which is available to emergency medical personnel. Toni was always under the care of an individual who knew about her medical problems. Under these circumstances, I usually discuss the relative need for medical identification jewelry. For very young children, one could probably consider that the jewelry might be a choking hazard. However, jewelry could avert problems should the child unexpectedly be in the care of someone unfamiliar with her allergies. It would be a good habit for Toni to wear a bracelet or medallion because Toni's allergies would probably continue for years to come. For older children and teenagers, who are likely to be involved in independent play and activities, medical identification jewelry is a potentially lifesaving device. Many families choose to list specific foods their child is allergic to on medical identification jewelry. Or you could indicate "food allergy" or "food allergy including" and then list maybe one or two foods. In this way, the medical identification jewelry would not be viewed as a menu of unsafe foods that implied all other foods would be safe for your child to consume.

Activating Emergency Medical Services

In the event of a severe allergic reaction, or if epinephrine is administered, it is important to seek prompt medical attention. I would usually not advise taking your child to a doctor's office because the doctor might not have all the therapies available in an emergency department. Getting to the emergency room quickly, in a car or on foot, without summoning an ambulance, might save time if you live near an emergency room; however, if symptoms have progressed, treating your child might be difficult, unless another adult were available. Therefore, calling for an ambulance to transport a child to an emergency care center is the safest choice. In many locations, call the emergency access telephone number, such as 911, to request an ambulance.

In some locations, ambulances have epinephrine on board. However, not all ambulances may carry epinephrine; check your state or local practices. When calling 911, state that your child is experiencing a severe allergic reaction and has food allergies. Let the dispatcher know which medications have been administered and that your child may need epinephrine. This could prompt the dispatcher to send a higher-level ambulance with a paramedic, who would be more likely to have epinephrine and treatments for severe allergic reaction. For school or camp emergency action plans, it may be sensible to determine the closest and best location to transport your child and have on your written emergency care plan the numbers needed to activate those services. Practice what you would say on the telephone, and teach your child how to activate emergency medical services if he is able.

Carrying and Storing Medications

An important component of the emergency care plan and emergency action plan is to know where medications are located and that they have not expired, are stored safely, and are easily accessible. Many older children could keep their medications in a purse, clipped to a belt, or in a backpack, but it is safer to have the medications attached, in some way, to the child because if he is separated from his backpack, the medications would still be accessible. In school or at camp, clearly labeled medications should be stored in unlocked cabinets. The emergency action plan should be located where the person assigned to treat your child can reach it quickly and easily. Practice drills for an emergency care plan should include accessing the written action plan in the event of an allergic reaction.

In later chapters, we discuss how the emergency action plan and emergency care plan are tailored to fit the specific circumstances of schools, camps, daycare settings, and other locations where your child may not be with you. In these situations, it is important to review, with all of the persons involved, how to keep your child safe. This truly requires a partnership of your child in an age-appropriate way, you, and those who care for your child. These plans should be initiated with the help of your physician. Consult your pediatrician or allergist to ensure that all pieces are in place in a way that is appropriate for your child's specific allergies. Everyone involved in your child's care should understand the basics of recognizing an allergic reaction and using the medications that have been described in this chapter. In Part 4, we consider another major component of the care plan for a food allergy, namely, avoiding food allergens.

PART 4

AVOIDING FOOD ALLERGENS

The treatment for a food allergy is to avoid the problem foods. This sounds simple but successfully avoiding a food allergen requires diligence in many settings where food will be acquired. Not infrequently, food proteins can end up in unexpected places, such as in vaccines or in medications.

Vaccines and Food Allergens

Many childhood vaccines exist, and all of these vaccines have possible allergic reactions as a side effect of their administration. These vaccines contain ingredients such as preservatives or antibiotics that may trigger an allergic reaction. However, two common proteins are found in vaccines and may be problematic for individuals with a food allergy. The first protein is egg.

Some "live" vaccines, where the virus used for the vaccine is alive but weakened, are grown in chicken egg embryos and, because of this processing, may carry with them some amount of egg protein in the final injection. Probably, the most famous childhood vaccine for which this has been an issue is the measles, mumps, and rubella (MMR) vaccination. Although this vaccine is grown in chicken egg embryos, various studies have found the amount of egg protein in the vaccine to be inconsequential and that even children with an anaphylactic egg allergy are not *significantly at risk of having an allergic reaction. The American Academy of Pediatrics' guidelines to infectious diseases and vaccination, called "The Red Book," indicates that the presence of an egg allergy is not a reason to be concerned about the administration of the MMR vaccine. Despite this recommendation, the package insert carries an egg allergy warning. I caution my patients that even though they may not be at any increased risk of having an allergic reaction to the MMR vaccine because of an egg allergy, an allergic reaction is still possible for any vaccine.*

In contrast to the MMR vaccine, two vaccines produced in chicken egg embryo may carry significant amounts of egg protein. The yellow fever vaccine is rarely administered. If you and your child were to travel to a country where yellow fever is found, such as sub-Saharan Africa, ask your allergist about receiving the vaccine in multiple small injections, even if your child has an anaphylactic allergy to egg. The influenza vaccine, a common vaccine, contains egg protein. This vaccine is given yearly and is formulated each year to treat a particular flu expected for that year. Recommendations for who should receive the influenza vaccine may change each year. You should discuss with your physician whether your child is a candidate for the vaccine. You should check with your pediatrician and allergist to determine whether an egg-free substitute for the flu vaccine is available. However, if no substitute is available, an egg-containing influenza vaccine is not generally recommended for individuals with an anaphylactic egg allergy.

The recommendation to avoid the influenza vaccine with egg protein raises several concerns. What determines an anaphylactic egg allergy? For example, for an individual who has ingested egg on several occasions and only had mild allergic reactions, would that person qualify as having an anaphylactic egg allergy? Would a child who has tested positive for egg allergy, yet has not eaten egg be considered at high risk for a reaction to the vaccine? Unfortunately, we do not have perfect answers to these questions. If I have diagnosed a definitive egg allergy in a child who must avoid egg protein, then I have to assume that the child could potentially have an anaphylactic egg allergy. In a study of individuals with a significant egg allergy, the influenza vaccine was administered in two injections instead of one. A small amount was given for the first injection, and the second injection contained the remainder of the vaccine. In that particular study, the children with egg allergies had no significant reaction. Perhaps the amount of egg in the vaccine should not be a concern. However, the amount of egg protein in the vaccine in that study was lower than the average amount found in vaccines in the years after the study. Also, the amount of egg protein in vaccines may vary by lot and manufacturer. It is difficult to know how much egg protein may be in any particular vaccine. Some manufacturers are now reporting the amount of egg in their vaccine, which may help allergists to evaluate vaccination risks.

Allergists may administer the flu vaccine, in small increments, to children with egg allergy if the child is at a high risk of significant illness should she catch the flu. For example, a child with serious asthma, lung damage, or cystic fibrosis could become very ill should she catch the flu. The risk of the vaccine (an allergic reaction) is weighed against the benefit of the vaccine's protection against influenza. Allergy skin tests of the vaccine may help determine part of the risk; if the tests are small or negative, there may be less risk. By discussing your child's situation with your allergist, you should be able to determine the best course of action. If vaccination cannot be performed, other options such as medicine to treat the flu are available.

Another food protein in vaccines is gelatin. The presence of gelatin is more complicated than the presence of egg in vaccines. You can read more about gelatin allergy in Chapter 8. Gelatin is used as a stabilizer in a variety of vaccines, although in very low doses in vaccines in the United States. Much of the gelatin used in U.S. vaccines has been processed to some degree and is possibly less allergenic. Gelatin can be found in vaccines for diphtheria, tetanus, and pertussis; influenza; Japanese encephalitis; measles, mumps, and rubella; typhoid; varicella (chicken pox), and yellow fever. Discuss your child's gelatin allergy with your allergist. The allergist may determine that, even though your child has a severe gelatin allergy, testing and a gradual administration of the vaccine may be an option; or versions of the vaccine with less gelatin might be an option.

Food Allergens in Medications

The same diligence you apply to reading labels and asking questions when acquiring foods for your food-allergic child is needed to scrutinize prescription and over-the-counter medications. Never assume that the prescribing doctor has already considered your child's food allergy when medications are prescribed. You should discuss your child's food allergies with your doctor and the pharmacist and whether any of the ingredients in a particular medication may be a problem.

Lactose is a milk sugar derived from milk, and pharmaceutical-grade lactose has generally been considered unlikely to contain any milk proteins. However, some recent studies have disclosed that lactose sometimes has a small amount of milk protein contamination. For example, lactose is used in some dry-powder asthma inhalers, and some children with a severe milk allergy may possibly react to the inhalation of the lactose in these inhalers. You should discuss this possibility with your pediatrician or allergist because non-lactose-containing inhalers can be substituted. Casein, a cow-milk protein, has some-

times been used as an anti-stick protein on latex gloves, another possibly unexpected source of milk protein to mention to your child's doctor or dentist.

If your child is undergoing surgery and will require anesthetics, you should certainly disclose his food allergies to the anesthesiologist and surgeon and remind them to check any medications and anesthetics for food proteins. Each of the drugs used by physicians include a comprehensive product or package insert that describes the medications' ingredients and often will include warnings about possible allergic reactions. For example, anesthetic agents may contain a small amount of egg protein that may be of concern if your child has an egg allergy.

Some of the warning labels on medications have been the source of confusion, for example, for certain asthma inhalers. Certain inhalers contain soy lecithin, which is a fatty derivative of soy. Soy lecithin contains an extremely low amount of detectable soy protein, which allergists usually consider not significant for most individuals with a soy allergy. The product insert on some of these items indicates a contraindication for the use of products with soy lecithin if there is an allergy to soybean or peanut. Ask your doctor how concerned you should be about this warning. Would the amount inhaled through these products likely cause an allergic reaction? One could also ask what the warning has to do with peanut, when the protein in question is actually from soy. Although there is no easy answer to this labeling contraindication for these products, many allergists will individualize the use of these medications, considering the risks and benefits for a particular child.

Hospitals

You might expect that food served in a hospital would be safe for your child as long as the hospital knows about your child's food allergies. Unfortunately, this is often not the case. It may be embarrassing for a physician to admit, but hospital food services may not be safe for children with food allergies, particularly those with multiple food allergies. Approach hospital meals as you would a restaurant meal (see Chapter 21). Specifically, you would disclose your child's food allergies to the hospital staff. Speak with hospital dietary services to review your child's specific food allergies. If there is an elective hospital admission for your child, you could do this possibly in advance of the hospital stay. You might request that a specific person in the dietary area be assigned to prepare and deliver your child's safe meals.

In Part 4, I consider the degree, or strictness, of avoidance that is necessary to keep your child safe. I discuss the amount of food that may cause an allergic reaction and also the problem of exposures through ingestion, skin contact, or inhalation. The avoidance of multiple foods can have potential nutritional consequences. The types of nutritional deficiencies that may be encountered during avoidance diets are discussed, as well as ways to avoid nutritional deficiencies and maintain a healthy diet for your child.

Because of many wonderful organizations, in particular the Food Allergy & Anaphylaxis Network, a lay organization with nearly thirty thousand members, and the work of many individuals and groups, families have access to resources to help plan diets for their children. Excellent information is available for how to purchase prepackaged foods, acquire restaurant meals, and approach a food allergy in school, at camp, and while traveling. Still parents are concerned about keeping their child safe in these environments. We will review the approaches needed to keep your child safe, and we will also consider common pitfalls and other issues. Understanding these issues will help you to provide a safe environment for your child and will give you the tools necessary to teach your child and others.

17 ~ Avoidance Diets

Two-year-old Pauline had experienced allergic reactions to eggs and milk. She was initially breast-fed, but when she was given yogurt at age 8 months, she developed hives. She had two other allergic reactions to milk and also experienced two allergic reactions to egg. Yogurt, cheese, French toast, and scrambled eggs triggered allergic reactions too. However, her family continued to give Pauline cookies and cakes that had egg or milk baked into them, and they did not notice any problems. Although a small taste of cheese pizza once caused hives, Pauline was able to tolerate breads baked with milk or butter. When I evaluated her, she had experienced allergic reactions to both milk and eggs within the previous six months. Her allergy tests indicated that she was at risk of reacting to milk and eggs. Pauline's family wondered whether it would be safe for her to eat baked foods containing eggs and milk, which she seemingly tolerated.

Strict versus Less Strict Avoidance

Some children with milk or egg allergy react to even small amounts of egg or milk baked into products. We certainly also see children who tolerate these foods without any apparent problem even though they have a reaction to larger amounts. If Pauline were experiencing chronic skin or gastrointestinal problems, I might have been more concerned, but she did not have these problems. Her family was taking two possible risks. One risk was that the amount of milk or egg in any given product they gave Pauline to eat would be unknown. I could not tell them what amount might trigger a reaction. At some point, however, some amount of milk or egg would cause a reaction.

Indeed, she had reacted to products containing whole milk or whole egg. Some children tolerate small amounts of milk or egg baked into the food. These amounts are probably tolerated for two reasons. First, the quantity of egg or milk in these baked products is low, and second, the heating from baking the food may break down some of the protein. These circumstances are *very* different from, say, cheese baked in food or eggs in French toast. The family would have to decide whether they were willing to take the risks.

The second risk is whether allowing Pauline to ingest these small amounts of egg and milk would affect her ability to outgrow these allergies in the long run. One school of thought suggests that through strict avoidance of the food the immune system may "forget" about the allergy and tolerate the food at a later time. Another school of thought argues that a small amount of exposure may help the immune system to learn to accept the food. Studies are under way to address these questions. It is unknown whether these exposures could speed, hinder, or have no effect on Pauline's eventually outgrowing the food allergy. Some families do not know whether their child could tolerate egg or milk baked into products. No simple blood or skin test can be performed to determine whether a particular child would tolerate this amount of exposure. Do not try to give your egg- or milk-allergic child these foods unless advised by your doctor.

The Amount of Food That May Trigger a Reaction

Most children with a diagnosed food allergy are instructed to strictly avoid the food. The primary reason to avoid the food is to avoid a reaction. Whether an occasional accidental ingestion of the avoided food hinders the ability to outgrow an allergy is not known. Although there are no comprehensive studies on this question, we do not believe, for example, that performing an oral food challenge hinders a child's chance to outgrow an allergy. More discussion about the effect of exposure to foods on the immune system can be found in Chapters 11 and 28.

It is natural to wonder how much of a particular food may trigger a reaction in your child. Unfortunately, no simple tests can tell how much food may trigger a reaction. You may expect that the larger the allergy skin test or the higher the food-specific IgE antibody in the bloodstream, the lesser the amount of food your child might tolerate. However, this is not necessarily the case. The amount of food that might trigger a reaction for a given individual is somewhat unpredictable, although some individuals are, on average, more sensitive than others. In studies that we conducted where food was given in gradually increasing amounts to children who had approximately a 50 percent chance of tolerating the food, the amount that triggered a reaction for half of the children was more than about a teaspoon of the food. However, one could ask, "What is the least amount of food that might trigger a reaction in my child?"

Only a modest number of studies have tried to determine the average amount of food that would provoke a significant reaction for an individual and also the amount of food that might provoke any degree of reaction for an individual. The more food ingested, the more likely a severe reaction will occur. This is why diagnostic oral food challenges are started with very low amounts of the food, and the amount eaten is gradually increased over time. In studies of individuals with peanut allergy, the amount of peanut that may typically bring on at least a mild reaction, for example, itchiness, is small. It is typically equivalent to somewhere between a fiftieth to one-half of a peanut kernel. However, the amount of peanut likely to cause a reaction that is stronger, for example, hives and vomiting, is about one-half of a peanut kernel or more. In studies of milk allergy, one or two drops have been known to cause a noticeable reaction in blinded challenges. However, many studies find a lowest-provoking dose of closer to one-half to one teaspoon of milk. Some children appear to be more sensitive and would have probably reacted to less than a drop of milk; this happens with egg too.

Not knowing how much of a particular food may trigger a reaction in your child can be frustrating. Also the theoretical concern exists that small amounts in the diet could be triggering the immune system to continue to attack the food. As mentioned previously, small exposures may "teach" the immune system to accept the food. We just do not know for certain whether such exposures are good, bad, or irrelevant, and the answer may vary depending on the child. Discuss with your doctor your child's past experiences with any reactions to foods to consider whether your child may be reactive to trace amounts of the food.

Some children tolerate larger or smaller amounts of the foods before they begin to have a reaction. To avoid any serious reactions, a strict avoidance diet is recommended. While strictly avoiding peanuts, tree nuts, and seafood is often suggested because these foods can cause severe reactions possibly triggered by trace amounts, there may be more leeway for individuals like Pauline who can tolerate baked goods that contain egg or milk. This also holds true for individuals who experience only an itchy mouth or milder symptoms from certain raw fruits and vegetables. Your doctor may individualize your child's avoidance for these reasons. Because studies that look at the effect of these various exposures are ongoing, you should request the most up-to-date information from your doctor.

Exposure through Skin Contact and Inhalation

Three-year-old Lyle was diagnosed with a milk allergy during infancy. His family came to my office because Lyle developed hives and wheezing while his mother was holding him as she prepared hot chocolate. The reaction occurred while Lyle was near the boiling hot chocolate. The milk protein became airborne during cooking, which triggered his reaction. The family was concerned that he was becoming more allergic to milk.

Food allergens can become airborne. We have undertaken research studies concerning peanut butter, an oily substance. We and other groups were not able to detect peanut protein around peanut butter, and when individuals with a peanut allergy sniffed peanut butter, they did not have any reactions. However, the literature does have cases about children who react to airborne foods. Some of these studies were described in Chapter 5 about food allergy and asthma. In the case of rapidly boiling hot chocolate or milk, the steam can carry the proteins. Scrambling eggs, frying fish, or boiling hot dogs can also create airborne proteins. Studies describe people who have reactions in fish markets where fish protein is abundant. In certain occupational settings such as bakeries or food-processing factories where wheat and powdered eggs are used, individuals can develop allergic reactions from the airborne foods. In general, the reactions are similar to what might be expected from other airborne proteins such as cat dander or pollens. For individuals with asthma, these exposures may trigger an asthmatic reaction, and for those who do not have asthma, hay fever symptoms, with itchy, running nose and red eyes, may result. If there is enough contact on the skin, as was the case for Lyle, there may also be rashes.

In general, children with significant food allergies should not be close to the foods to which they are allergic when those foods are being cooked. Powdery foods, such as powdered milk and wheat flour, become airborne easily; therefore, when you are cooking with these products, it seems prudent to do so when your child is not nearby. The severity of reactions from airborne food proteins may not be any worse than might be expected from exposure to nonfood airborne allergens, such as animal dander or pollens, but it seems that avoidance in these special circumstances is sensible.

Lyle's family was also concerned about skin contact with the foods to which he was allergic, especially milk. I described for Lyle's family the study

IN DEPTH ON UNUSUAL FOOD EXPOSURES

Your child could be exposed to a food protein in many unexpected ways. Many of these exposures are minor because they involve skin contact and would not be expected to result in anaphylaxis. However, some exposures include ingestion and could cause more severe reactions.

Kissing

If an individual without food allergies had eaten a meal that included a particular food allergen and then passionately kissed someone sensitive to that food, saliva containing the allergen would have been transferred by mouth. This exposure could result in significant allergic reactions. Studies have shown that among adults with food allergies, about 1 in 20 have experienced allergic reactions from passionate kissing. In contrast, reactions from a casual kiss, for example, a kiss on the cheek, is less likely to cause a severe reaction.

Kissing is a concern for teenagers and young adults with food allergies. For these children, clear warnings about passionate kissing must be emphasized. In studies that my team and others have undertaken, brushing the teeth after a meal could be insufficient for removing the allergen from the mouth. Although not foolproof, our studies using peanut butter showed that avoiding ingesting the allergen for a number of hours and then ingesting a meal that does not contain the allergen, possibly along with brushing the teeth, would greatly reduce the risk. However, it is best for the partner not to eat the allergen in the first place. A trusted partner will usually comply.

Other Intimate Contact

When an individual without food allergies ingests a food protein, that protein can reach the bloodstream and circulate throughout the body in an allergenic form. Can this protein emerge in sweat or other bodily fluids such as semen? I am unaware of any reports of allergic responses from sweat, and it seems physiologically unlikely that significant proteins from foods would emerge in the sweat. It has been difficult to detect any food proteins in semen, but one study reported this as a concern in one individual. It seems that this is not a common occurrence, probably for two reasons. The amount of food protein in semen is probably too low to cause a reaction for most people, and the concerned partner probably avoids the allergen when intimate contact, for example, kissing, is expected, which reduces the risk of exposing a partner to the allergen.

Participation in Sports

Children may not expect to be exposed to food allergens when participating in sports, and our studies have disclosed that teenagers often neglect to bring their emergency medications to sporting events. They do not expect to eat while playing sports so they do not perceive a risk. However, exposure to a food allergen during a sporting event is possible. For example, individuals may be prone to passing around drinks. If someone has eaten a food your child is allergic to, drank from a straw or a cup, and then passed the drink to your child, the cup or straw might carry the allergen. In addition, snacks are often provided at sporting events. Emphasize to your child that sharing straws, cups, and utensils can pose a danger and should be avoided. Coaches should be aware of food allergies, treatment should be available on site, and medical alert jewelry should be worn.

Blood Transfusion

Because ingested food proteins can make their way into the bloodstream, a person donating blood may be passing on some of the food proteins they have ingested. Should you worry about these food proteins if your child required a blood transfusion? Calculations have been made on the potential amount of food protein that could be transferred in a blood transfusion. In a blood transfusion, the liquid part of the blood is separated from the red blood cells. Usually, the red blood cells are transfused into the person who is receiving the blood transfusion. The amount of a food protein that would be present in the liquid part of the blood donation would be exceptionally small and unlikely to trigger a reaction. Because most of this liquid is removed, residual food proteins in the transfusion of red blood cells are further reduced. In cases in which an allergic child receives a blood transfusion, he would be under medical care and monitored for any reaction, so several levels of protection would be in place. If your child is having elective surgery and requiring a directed blood donation by a known blood donor, for added safety ask the person to avoid foods your child is allergic to for twelve to twenty-four hours before the transfusion.

Cosmetics

Hundreds of skin-care and cosmetic products on the market specifically include food proteins as ingredients. Many of these products advertise these food proteins. Before purchasing shampoos, conditioners, moisturizers, or cosmetics, read the ingredients in case these products contain food allergens. In some cases, the manufacturer may need to be contacted to determine the specific ingredients because laws that cover foods do not cover these cosmetic products. Ask the manufacturer whether particular allergens may be present in the item. Discuss with your doctor the possibility of applying a small amount of the item to an area of the skin before using the product on larger areas. Of course, it is possible to have allergic reactions to nonfood ingredients in cosmetics and creams.

Alcoholic Beverages

I hope most of the children with food allergies you care for, and who are presumably under the legal drinking age, are not routinely ingesting alcoholic beverages! However, it is important to know that certain alcoholic beverages may contain food allergens. Some individuals have a metabolic disorder and cannot process alcohol normally. They may develop a variety of allergy-like symptoms from ingesting an alcoholic beverage. An individual may have an allergic reaction to the primary ingredients in that beverage. For example, some individuals may be allergic to the grains used to make beer. Some alcoholic beverages use clarifying agents that have perhaps unexpected proteins in them, such as egg or fish proteins. The allergic potential of the final product in regard to egg or fish allergy has not been extensively studied, and there are no reports in the literature of significant allergic reactions in adults regarding these items, but you should be aware of them. Some liqueurs may contain nut proteins. So read the labels and contact manufacturers as needed.

Alcohol may speed the absorption of food allergens. A food that might have caused a mild reaction or no reaction on its own could cause a more significant reaction when ingested along with alcohol. Alcohol can impair judgment. A teenager who drinks alcohol may make wrong food choices. Discuss the ramifications of alcohol and food allergies with your child.

Items Not Usually or Often Eaten

Squirrels, not people, usually eat acorns. No reports document allergy to acorns, even though I suspect acorns could be an allergen. Casual exposure to acorns in the outdoors, assuming they are not eaten, would not usually cause concern. Of course, if you have a young child with multiple nut allergies, she should be kept away from acorns (though choking is probably a stronger concern than allergy). Otherwise, it seems prudent to remind your child not to eat the acorns. There may be other food items that your allergic child would usually not have the opportunity to eat, such as less common seeds (e.g., pumpkin) or very exotic fruits or nuts. Typically, there is at least some potential for an allergy to these foods, and you should discuss these issues with your doctor before trying them. Modeling dough used in play could contain wheat ingredients. Though the product is not meant to be eaten, it could cause skin reactions in a child with wheat allergy.

that we conducted in which a pea-sized amount of peanut butter was placed on the skin for a minute and then wiped away. Thirty highly peanut-allergic children who underwent this procedure had no symptoms beyond the area where the peanut butter was placed. Only a third of the children had redness or swelling in that area, and two-thirds had no symptoms. I explained that we routinely perform allergy skin tests with a variety of foods. The food is scratched onto the skin; yet, it is highly unusual to see serious reactions from this type of exposure. Certain circumstances occur where skin contact is more of an issue because large areas of skin are exposed or the areas exposed are not intact. For example, many cosmetic products or skin-care products contain food proteins, and spreading these over the body could cause a rash or reaction. In particular, if a cream or ointment that contains a food protein is spread on abraded, scratched skin of a child with severe atopic dermatitis, it would be easier for the food proteins to seep into the body because the usual skin barrier is broken. If a child has widespread eczema and were to be splashed or soaked in a larger amount of a food to which he or she is allergic, there might be more severe reactions than just flares of skin rashes. Many skin-care or hair-care products may contain nut oils or other food proteins that should be avoided for these reasons.

With airborne proteins and skin contact, there are also theoretical concerns about increasing the body's immune response to food allergens (described in Chapter 28). Use prudence when foods are cooking. Read ingredient labels carefully, especially for products used on the skin.

~

When your doctor has diagnosed a food allergy in your child, a strict avoidance diet is typically recommended. Occasionally, small amounts of an allergenic food such as eggs or milk baked into a food may be allowed into the diet if you understand the risks involved and are willing to take them; research on this situation is incomplete, so talk to your allergist first. Trace amounts of an ingested allergen may pose a risk of an allergic reaction for some individuals. There are no simple tests to determine how much food may trigger a reaction for your child, but some children are sensitive to trace amounts, while the average allergic child may be more likely to react to modest amounts often in excess of a teaspoon. Casual exposure by airborne or skin contact is unlikely to cause a severe allergic reaction, but it could pose a concern in certain settings such as during cooking or if there were widespread skin contact.

18 ~ Maintaining a Nutritious Diet

Beth was an underweight 1-year-old whose family brought her to my office to be evaluated for food allergies. She had severe eczema. She was also experiencing occasional vomiting and diarrhea. The family had indicated infant formula that contained milk resulted in a significant increase in her symptoms, so they were trying other formulas. A nutritionist recommended a soy-based protein drink. The soy-based protein drink did not contain the vitamins and minerals she would need to grow. Supplemental vitamins were crushed into powder and added to the soy protein drink. But Beth continued to do poorly and did not gain weight. Beth's diet consisted of the soy protein drink and eight types of vitamins and supplements mixed into the soy drink. The rest of Beth's diet was limited to a few fruits and vegetables.

Although I am an allergist and not a trained dietitian, I reviewed some of the components of Beth's current diet and saw that not much fat was provided. The soy drink was formulated for adults who do not require as much as infants. In addition, Beth had not undergone a prior evaluation for food allergy, and many of her symptoms were clearly associated with food allergies. It was likely that components of her current diet were causing a problem. Indeed, Beth was allergic to soy, the major protein in her diet. I suggested that the family switch to a commercial infant formula, even though Beth was already 1 year old. These are complete formulas that contain the nutrients needed to support growth. In addition, we could provide Beth with a hypoallergenic formula for children with milk or soy allergy, an extensive hydrolysate, casein-based formula. Because most children with milk allergy tolerate this type of formula, it would be a convenient source of nutrition for Beth. Her family would no longer need to use numerous vitamin and mineral supplements, and they would have a primary source of nutrition for Beth. Beth did extremely well on the infant formula and began to gain weight, and we were able to add other foods to her diet based on the results of additional testing.

Beth's story is unfortunate because her initial evaluations did not consider the possibility that she was ingesting a food she was allergic to. At the same time, the nutritionist did not appreciate the nutritional needs of an infant and was not providing adequate nutrients for proper growth and development. For any child diagnosed with food allergies for which several common foods are being removed from the diet, nutritional concerns certainly arise. A child on a restricted diet must be carefully monitored for growth, and the diet must be reviewed for nutritional adequacy. Of course, the more foods restricted from the diet, the more concerns there would be about nutritional issues.

Assuming that a child with food allergy is otherwise healthy and has no increased nutritional requirements because of a chronic illness such as eczema or intestinal problems, the nutritional requirements would be similar to those of children who have no food allergies. The primary components of a healthy diet include protein, fat, carbohydrates, vitamins, minerals, and trace elements. Caloric intake, the amount of energy from the diet, is an important consideration for proper growth and development. Calories are derived from the intake of protein, fat, and carbohydrates. Caloric needs change as children grow and also vary among boys and girls. In addition to energy, specific nutrients in the diet are needed to ensure proper body functions and to prevent illness. Proteins are a source of amino acids, the building blocks of life. Good-quality proteins that include specific, much-needed essential amino acids are typically obtained from meats or complementary foods, such as classic rice and beans. Fats are an important source of calories, and essential fatty acids (linoleic and linolenic) are necessary for proper brain development in infants. These types of essential fatty acids are found in fish, which is often excluded from the diet of an individual with food allergy. However, essential fatty acids are also available in vegetable oil such as canola, corn, soy, and olive. The diet should consist of a blend of saturated fats, which are usually obtained from animal origin but also from monosaturated and polyunsaturated fats, which are components of vegetable oils such as safflower, canola, corn, soy, and olive. Carbohydrates or complex sugars are a major source of calories needed for growth and generally account for nearly half of the caloric intake. Vegetables, fruits, and grains contain carbohydrates. Wheat products are a common source of carbohydrates. However, this food may often be restricted for a child with food allergy. Substitutions for carbohydrates could, therefore, include rice, oat, potato, corn, or quinoa.

Vitamins, minerals, and trace elements are necessary for the normal function of various parts of the body such as blood clotting, bone development, teeth development, and nerve and muscle function. For example, vitamin A helps with growth and night vision, and vitamin D aids the body's use of calcium. Examples of minerals include calcium for bone development and iron for the blood. Trace elements in the body include zinc, which is important for healing and immune function.

Specific Considerations in an Allergen-Restricted Diet

When a child's diet excludes milk, egg, wheat, soy, peanut, tree nuts, fish, and shellfish, less allergenic foods that maintain a balanced, nutritious diet should be substituted. The first consideration would be to maintain appropriate amounts of protein, fat, and carbohydrate in the diet. For protein, one or two servings of meat each day would usually suffice, but more servings could be recommended for already restricted diets. Many meats include fat, but to ensure that essential fatty acids are included, vegetable oils, such as canola, corn, soy, or olive oil, could be added to meats or other foods. With a wheat-free diet, alternative grains, fruits, and vegetables can be substituted and, perhaps, rice, oat, potato, or corn can be included in the diet. Young children like Beth could be provided with a complete formula, but older children, if they are unable to maintain the major portions of their diet from the allowed foods, may also require a nutritionally balanced supplemental formula. For example, individuals who are on highly restricted elimination or elemental diets, where there are only a few foods for them to ingest, would need, for example, an amino acid–based formula that contains all the various nutrients required for proper growth and development. This type of formula is sometimes also used as a "backup" when an individual's diet only includes limited foods. Ideally, children on such restricted diets would undergo evaluations to ensure that additional calorie-, protein-, fat-, and carbohydrate-enriched foods would be available. When selecting particular foods, it may be possible to obtain vitamin-, mineral-, and trace element–enriched versions of the foods such as infant cereals.

When major allergens are removed from the diet, certain vitamins and minerals may also be reduced. The following list shows vitamins and minerals that are components of major food allergens and a list of alternative sources that are less allergenic. The amount of nutrient in the alternative sources may vary greatly. For example, a calcium-fortified soy drink may or have ounce-for-ounce calcium levels similar to milk, and a calcium-fortified beverage likely has much more calcium per serving than a vegetable. Be sure to discuss these substitutions with your doctor and/or dietitian.

Nutrient	*Allergen*	*Alternative sources*
Vitamin A	Milk	Spinach, potato, squash, carrot
Vitamin D	Milk	Fortified alternative "milks" and juices, margarine
Vitamin E	Peanut	Green leafy vegetables, vegetable oils, grains
Thiamin	Soy, wheat	Pork, beef, beans, grains
Riboflavin	Milk, egg, soy, wheat	Meats, leafy green vegetables, grains
Niacin	Wheat, peanut	Meats, beans, enriched grains
Vitamin B12	Milk, egg	Meats
Folate	Soy	Leafy green vegetables, beans
Pantothenic acid	Milk, egg	Meats, fruits, vegetables, grains
Calcium	Milk	Leafy green vegetables, beans, calcium-fortified drinks
Chromium	Peanut	Whole grains
Iron	Wheat, soy	Meat, beans, dried fruits, iron-fortified grains
Magnesium	Soy, peanut	Fruits, vegetables, grains
Manganese	Peanut	Leafy green vegetables, whole grains
Phosphorus	Milk, soy	Poultry meats, carbonated beverages
Selenium	Egg	Meat, grains
Zinc	Soy	Meat, beans

Among the various nutrients that may be deficient in an allergen-restricted diet, one study shows that calcium, iron, vitamin D, vitamin E, and zinc were being obtained at less than recommended amounts in the diet of children with food allergies. Of course, additional diet restrictions, such as vegetarian, gluten-free, or low-sugar diets, may need to be addressed. Family preferences or other medical illnesses may impose additional nutritional concerns.

Families undertaking restrictive diets might face significant pitfalls. Because children with multiple food allergies often tolerate rice, rice drinks often become a major component of the diet. Unfortunately, these are low in protein, and alternative sources of protein should be considered if rice drinks are used. Children on a milk-restricted diet may receive too little calcium, so calcium-fortified juices and soy or rice drinks should be kept on hand. However, the calcium-fortified juices may have less calcium than the fortified rice and soy drinks. Calcium supplement tablets may need to be added to the diet.

If your child is only avoiding one or two foods, but the diet is otherwise well rounded, and any major nutrient, such as calcium in a milk-restricted diet, are being provided adequately, then it is unlikely that any nutritional problems will develop. However, if more than a few foods have been eliminated from your child's diet, or if your child is not growing as expected, then talk to your pediatrician and consider an evaluation from a registered pediatric dietitian. Resources for obtaining a dietitian are listed in Part 9. Typically, a three- to seven-day diet record would be obtained. Your dietitian can evaluate this diet record to determine whether your child is obtaining the appropriate calories and balance of protein, carbohydrate, fats, vitamins, minerals, and trace elements needed for proper growth and development. If there are potential deficiencies, substitutions could be suggested, such as using additional oils or taking multivitamins, iron, or calcium. Of course, it is vital to review your child's specific food allergies with your dietitian, so the substitute foods are appropriately selected. Obviously, the material in this chapter is not comprehensive for you to rely on solely for ensuring that your child has a healthy diet. You should discuss the particular aspects of your child's diet with your allergist, pediatrician, and possibly dietitian.

Children who are on food elimination diets may be at risk for caloric deficiency or deficiencies of particular components of the diet, such as essential fats, amino acids or protein, carbohydrates, and important vitamins, minerals, and trace elements. If only a few foods have been eliminated from the diet, simple substitution foods that provide adequate nutrition can be given. However, wide elimination diets may require the use of supplemental complete formulas to provide the needed nutrients. Expert guidance by a pediatric dietitian may be necessary. Brief elimination trial diets, for example, one or two weeks, used to diagnose food allergy, are unlikely to have an adverse effect on long-term growth or development and would require less concern about substitutions and evaluations.

19 ~ Navigating the Supermarket

Billy is a 5-year-old who has milk allergy and loves ham. As a treat, his mother would allow him to have a few slices of ham in the supermarket. Billy had eaten ham from the supermarket two dozen times. However, on this particular day, Billy began to cry as he was eating the slices of ham. His mother noticed that he had hives and was coughing. She gave him his emergency medications and, instead of driving home, drove several blocks to a local emergency room. Billy did fine, but what had caused this allergic reaction? Even though his mother had purchased ham from this deli counter many times without a problem, it was very likely that the slicer used for the ham had been contaminated with milk protein from cheese that was previously sliced on the machine. Billy's mother confronted the deli staff, and they confirmed that cross-contact was likely. Billy's mother no longer purchases store-sliced ham. However, she still treats Billy to sliced ham from a safe, labeled package obtained from a commercial supplier.

The supermarket may seem like a minefield. The prepared foods section and deli counters could be highly prone to contact with allergens from other foods. Manufactured packaged products on grocery shelves that contain ingredient labels are potentially safer but require diligent label reading and a knowledge about labeling practices. This chapter will consider some of the pitfalls in supermarket shopping. Understanding some of these pitfalls will help you shop more safely for your child. We will also explore the benefits and limitations of the new labeling laws that require the identification of major allergens. Finally, we will consider some of the ambiguities in current labeling practices and how they affect your ability to obtain safe foods. With this knowledge, obtaining safe, manufactured packaged foods for your child should be a less stressful and safer experience.

Pitfalls in Obtaining Safe Packaged Products

Before the new labeling laws, manufacturers were not required to list in plain English the allergenic foods in their products. For example, the term *casein* would be used without using the term *milk*. Only well-informed families would know that casein is indeed milk protein. We analyzed telephone calls made to the Food Allergy & Anaphylaxis Network, where members voluntarily disclosed their experiences with food labeling. Our study revealed that companies may switch ingredients in their products without obvious notification. Different sizes of the same item may have different ingredients. Some packaged products contain a label on the outer wrapper, but the items inside each have their own labels that may differ from the outside label. All ingredient labels should be read each time a particular food is purchased; do not make any assumptions.

Sometimes ingredient labels contain errors. In studies we conducted with the Food Allergy & Anaphylaxis Network, and also in studies that were reported by the U.S. Food and Drug Administration (FDA), we found that companies sometimes, in error, prepare food that contains an allergen without listing the ingredient on the label. These pitfalls are surmountable. Smaller bakeries and confectioneries may have a higher risk of including peanuts, eggs, milk, or nuts in their products without disclosing these ingredients on labels, unless they are specifically allergy-aware. The FDA found that about 25 percent of confectionery or bakery companies had errors in their labeling. Inspections and better label regulations have corrected many of these problems in the recent years.

We conducted a study in which families were asked to read labels and to identify labels listing the food or ingredient they need to avoid. Only 10 percent of the families correctly identified all of the labels that listed milk, 25 percent identified soy, 50 percent peanut, and 90 percent accurately identified wheat and egg. New labeling laws that require obvious disclosure of allergens could reduce errors; yet, some of the errors occurred because families did not look at the various locations on the labels that indicated particular ingredients in the product. The lesson here is to read each label carefully and completely.

FALCPA

The Food Allergen Labeling and Consumer Protection Act of 2004 (FALCPA) took effect January 2006. The law requires that the eight major allergens or allergenic food groups—milk, egg, fish, shellfish, tree nuts, wheat, peanuts, and soy—be declared on ingredient labels using plain English. No longer would words such as "casein" or "whey" be sufficient. Although nearly two hundred foods have been identified to cause allergic reactions, these eight foods and food groups have been the primary focus of the legislation. Foods such as sesame and other seeds have not been included but are under consideration. The law applies to all types of packaged foods except for meat, eggs, poultry products, and raw agricultural foods such as fruits and vegetables in their natural state. The plain English words used to identify the foods may be placed within the ingredient list or as a separate "contains" statement. Before this law, the product might list "natural flavors." Now, the label may read "natural flavors (milk)" or may not mention milk within the ingredient statement but rather in a separate area of the label that says "contains milk." If the label says "natural flavor" but does not specify an allergen, the natural flavor might not be one of the recognized major allergens, but it still might be a food or ingredient your child avoids. The law does not exclude using more scientific terms for food allergens as long as the label indicates, in some location, the plain English term for the food. For example, the word "casein" may be used, but the word "milk" must also appear on the label. In addition, the law requires that the specific type of allergen be named. "Fish" or "shellfish" is not sufficient. Instead "salmon" or "lobster" would need to be named specifically. Terms such as "soybean," "soy," and "soya" are considered interchangeable. If the product has a "contains" statement, it is required that the "contains" statement list all of the major allergens that are in the food. The law took effect January 2006, and many products have a long shelf life, so it may take time for all products to reflect the labeling changes.

The FALCPA legislation is likely to reduce significantly accidental exposures to food allergens because using plain English terms and identifying major allergens rectified many of the pitfalls we identified in studies before the legislation. The legislation is a triumph of the work of parents, politicians, various government and industry groups, and organizations that advocate for food-allergic children, including the Food Allergy & Anaphylaxis Network and the Food Allergy Initiative.

The legislation has limitations. Only the eight major allergenic groups are considered. There are opportunities in the future for petitions from the public or health officials to request including additional foods if they are deemed to be of major consequence for consumers. For now, however, vague labeling such as "spices" or "natural flavoring" is still allowed.

The FALCPA legislation does not consider how much of a food protein in a given product may make it unsafe. This "threshold" issue is a double-edged sword. On the one hand, you may wish for your food to contain absolutely no trace of the food protein to which your child is allergic. On the other hand, it is difficult, in many cases, for manufacturers to be sure that none of a particular protein allergen remains. Before the law, processing aids such as soy lecithin were not declared on food labels. Soy lecithin is a fatty derivative of soy that contains a small amount of soy protein. The amount of soy protein in soy lecithin would likely not cause an allergic reaction for most people allergic to soy. Soy lecithin is used as an anti-stick agent in many baked products or it can be added directly to the food. You could imagine that if the soy lecithin has only touched the edge of a food and does not contain very significant amounts of soy protein to begin with, then the food should be safe for someone with soy allergy. However, the legislation does not differentiate, and a food product may be listed as "contains soy," even though most experts would believe the product is likely to be safe.

Indeed, the law acknowledges that certain forms of highly processed oils may not contain any appreciable protein and are exempt from labeling as an allergen. For example, soy oil is considered a highly refined oil that does not appear to be associated with allergic reactions, even though extremely low levels of protein may be detectable in soy oil when highly sensitive tests are used. Because the interpretation of these laws and possible additions or revisions to these laws are likely to change with time, I would urge you to look periodically for updates either through the Food Allergy & Anaphylaxis Network or from the Center for Food Safety and Applied Nutrition, a branch of the FDA (see Part 9).

Because the new labeling laws allow certain potential allergens to be in foods without special labeling (e.g., sesame) and include labeling for products with soy lecithin that you and your doctor may feel your child does not need to avoid, it may be necessary to contact manufacturers to get more information about ingredients in a particular product. Many manufacturers are forthcoming about the specific ingredients in their foods. For example, if your child is allergic to garlic or sesame, you may wish to contact the manufacturer to find out what "spices" have been used. When you call a manufacturer, identify yourself as a consumer with a child who has a food allergy and ask specifically about whether the product contains the ingredients your child is allergic to. Most companies will indicate whether the food you are asking about is in their product. However, they may be reluctant to tell you exactly which ingredients constitute natural flavoring or spices. They want to keep some of these ingredients secret, but they are usually willing to answer yes or no to specific food ingredients. In some cases, I have needed to intervene and write letters to the company. I have also signed nondisclosure agreements so that a manufacturer would let me know whether a particular allergen was in a food.

"May Contain" Labels

During a follow-up visit for the evaluation of a peanut allergy, Scott's family indicated that they had been giving him a particular snack food the entire previous year. They had just realized that the packaging warns "may contain peanut," the very food to which Scott is allergic. He had probably ingested this product fifty to one hundred times in the preceding year with no complaints. Was it safe for them to continue to give it to Scott? Indeed, the FALCPA legislation does not regulate the use of "may contain" statements. Companies have used these statements when a particular allergen is not an ingredient of the food but may have become a part of the food despite good manufacturing processes.

Companies are required to use care in ensuring that the ingredients listed on the product label accurately disclose what is in the product. However, you can imagine that during manufacturing, certain ingredients not meant to enter a product may accidentally cross-contact the food because of insufficient cleaning or unintentional spreading of an allergen within a factory. Numerous examples of reactions have occurred because of these errors. For example, milk-allergic children have reacted to apple juice packaged in cardboard juice boxes. The same equipment used to fill boxes with apple juice had been used to fill similar boxes with milk and so there was residual milk in the processing equipment. Even when manufacturers separate processing lines, some crossover could occur. For example, perhaps egg-free pasta is being made on one conveyor belt and egg pasta on another. In these or similar situations, companies could indicate "may contain" on the label. Since labeling for the possibility of allergen contact is voluntary, different words are sometimes used. Sometimes a company will indicate the food was "processed in a facility" with an allergen or "shared equipment" is used. Although one may presume the danger is stronger with a shared equipment rather than in a shared facility, it is difficult to know what the degree of risk truly is in either of these situations. Food-allergic consumers have become frustrated and think that perhaps these companies are simply pasting warnings on products to protect themselves, even when there is no true risk. However, it seems more likely that these companies are generally making a good faith effort to label their products as best as they can.

I understood Scott's parents' dilemma. Scott had eaten this product fifty to one hundred times with no problem. However, I do not work for the company that makes this product, and they may have a very good reason for putting the "may contain" label on the product. I advised that Scott stop eating this product. I encouraged Scott's family to contact the company to find out more about the label warning, and perhaps the company could consider ensuring that peanut would not be a part of the product that Scott has enjoyed. Some companies are responsive to requests from families and work harder to try to separate their equipment and to reduce the risks of cross-contact. If this can be achieved, it may be possible to eliminate the "may contain" warning. In the meantime, I suggest products labeled with provisional warnings should be avoided. Happily, a growing number of specialty companies, in particular confection and bakery companies, are specializing in allergy-safe packaged foods, which is increasing choices of safe packaged foods for families with children with food allergies.

~

For families with a child with food allergies, supermarket shopping is unfortunately time consuming and often frustrating. However, careful label reading each time an item is purchased is an important task. Because of stronger labeling laws, food labeling has improved, making it easier to find the major food allergens. Still, it is necessary to read the labels carefully each time a food is purchased. If your child is allergic to a food other than the "big eight" allergens or allergenic food groups, you will need to read particularly carefully, watching for terms that are not specific such as "natural flavors" and "spices." I hope studies under way to better determine the threshold, or lowest amounts of foods that may cause reactions, will allow companies to label foods without overexcluding ones that may be safe for your child.

In the meantime, there are several things that you can do to help ensure safety for your child and others. If you notice a problem with the label, notify the manufacturer and the FDA (see Part 9 for instructions on reporting). You may also wish to contact the Food Allergy & Anaphylaxis Network. Companies will often voluntarily recall products or make changes on labels in response to these reports. Read the label each time you purchase a product and involve your children in an age-appropriate way in helping to identify safe foods. Some online grocers are now showing ingredient labels on their Web sites and are including allergen ingredients. Although online grocers who deliver to your home may not be widely available, if they are, they may represent an additional convenience. Still, make sure you look at the label on the actual product that you receive to ensure that nothing has changed and the food is safe for your child. Finally, a growing number of specialty-food companies are creating allergen-free food products, adding additional convenience for shopping.

20 ~ At Home and in Social Settings

Four-year-old Donna had been diagnosed with peanut, tree nut, milk, and egg allergies before her first birthday. Her family decided that the best way to manage her multiple food allergies at home was to make their home free of the foods Donna was allergic to. For the past several years, her family had maintained every member of their household, which included Donna's older brother and also her grandmother, on the same allergen-free diet as Donna. The family found that trying to include the ingredients to which Donna was allergic in foods for the rest of the family led to pitfalls. For example, Donna would grab her older brother's food, or there would be confusion about which foods were safe for Donna.

In contrast to Donna's household, Ramsey's family did not exclude foods. Ramsey, a 5-year-old who was diagnosed with multiple food allergies before his first birthday, was allergic to egg, fish, shellfish, peanuts, and tree nuts. Ramsey's older brother and younger sister did not have food allergies and were allowed to eat the foods Ramsey could not. The family was careful to separate the foods that Ramsey was not allowed to consume from those that were safe for him. The family was careful not to have Ramsey in the kitchen while they were cooking fish or shellfish. They ensured that utensils used for the foods Ramsey was avoiding were not mixed with those that would be used with Ramsey's safe foods. Dishes and utensils were cleaned in typical ways that were adequate to remove food so Ramsey could use them safely. In Donna's home, where her older brother was restricted from many common foods, the family would treat her older brother to special meals in restaurants. In Ramsey's family, where Ramsey was restricted from eating foods that his younger sister and older brother were allowed to ingest, Ramsey was given special treats that were safe for him. Both families were satisfied with their approaches to keep their children safe and happy.

Families have many approaches to keep their homes safe for their food-allergic child. Many personal decisions must be made that consider all members of the family and the abilities of caregivers. Creating safe meals at home requires time and care to avoid accidental ingestions that occur through cross-contact exposures of the allergenic foods. Deciding to ban a food is easier but can have emotional consequences for the family. Eating safely at the homes of friends and relatives and providing safe meals for special occasions or parties are obstacles that also can be successfully surmounted with the right education and preparation. These will be the topics of this chapter.

Food Allergies at Home

Donna's family and Ramsey's family took very different approaches to provide safe meals for their children at home. I generally suggest to parents of food-allergic children to consider what they and their children enjoy eating and to discuss among the adults involved about the potential approaches. A decision to exclude particular foods from the home may depend on the types of foods involved. For example, having a peanut-free home may be more easily accomplished than having a milk-free home. Whether it is necessary to exclude a food from the home may depend on the perceived ease at which this can be accomplished and potential nutritional and emotional consequences for everyone involved. For example, if the food-allergic child is apt to grab other individual's food, it would be necessary to institute much more care if the food were maintained in the home. For example, keeping allergenic foods out of reach on higher shelves and strict supervision when a sibling is eating a food near the child with a food allergy may be a necessary and reasonable solution for some families.

Sometimes siblings are excellent at helping to protect their younger or older food-allergic sibling. In some circumstances, however, this may not be an additional safety net and may pose a source of danger, for example, when numerous siblings are eating the food that the child with allergies is expected to avoid. Families may choose to exclude highly allergenic foods that are not a staple of the diet. This usually includes peanut, tree nuts, fish, or shellfish. In my experience, not many families try to exclude egg, milk, wheat, or soy from the home. However, sometimes a family with young children finds it easier to restrict ubiquitous foods such as milk. This often comes up when twins are involved, where one has a food allergy and the other does not, and it is often easier to treat both with the same restrictive diet. As children get older, many families adjust the types of foods that they restrict from the home. For example, as Donna's family became comfortable that Donna was less likely to grab foods from others, they strongly considered returning milk and egg to the family diet. Theoretically, learning to live around a food in the home may be a good "life lesson" for later independence.

When families like Ramsey's have allergenic foods around the home, a variety of rules must be established to maintain safety for the child with food allergies. Ramsey was too young to know how to obtain safe foods on his own, and so he was taught to always ask whether he could eat a particular snack. He was also trusted not to share food with his siblings. Particular snacks that were safe for Ramsey were labeled with a green piece of tape as they were purchased or made at home. Containers used in the refrigerator or in storage areas in Ramsey's home were also labeled with green tape if they contained foods that were safe for Ramsey. Because several of the foods to which Ramsey was allergic would be cooked in the home, including egg, fish, and, on occasion, shellfish, these foods were prepared when Ramsey was not in the kitchen. Ramsey's parents knew that when they were preparing breakfast, lunch, or dinner, they would be careful with the utensils, countertop, and food preparation containers so as not to contaminate any of Ramsey's food. They typically would prepare Ramsey's meal first, before using foods to which he was allergic. When foods were stored in the refrigerator, they would always be enclosed in covered containers so that any spills within the refrigerator would not contaminate his foods. The family would occasionally have mealtime discussions about how they were continuing to keep Ramsey safe. This was particularly important because of Ramsey's younger sister. Ramsey was the one who had to be in charge of making sure that he did not take any foods from his younger sister.

Ramsey's family did make some mistakes and learned from them. Ramsey's father enjoyed cashew nuts and had been eating them in the living room of their home. He disposed of the packaging for the cashew nuts and wiped cashew crumbs off his shirt with a dishtowel. The next day, Ramsey washed his hands and face at the kitchen sink and used the same dishtowel to dry off. His eyes swelled and reddened, the residue from the nuts was on the dishtowel and caused this reaction. Ramsey's skin reaction was not severe, but it reminded his family that they had to be particularly clean and careful.

Many families compromise to help keep everyone safe. Ramsey's family had found a number of ways to make it possible for family members to continue to enjoy the foods Ramsey was allergic to, while Donna's family found it easier to have everyone avoid the allergenic foods. Both families continued to have open discussions about ways to enjoy nutritious meals and still maintain safety for their children.

Relatives and Family Gatherings

Denise is a 9-year-old with a peanut allergy whose family typically provided all of her meals when Denise ate outside of the home, or they helped Denise order a safe meal in a restaurant. Denise's grandmother felt that she too could provide Denise with meals that were safe. While Denise was at her grandmother's home, her grandmother offered her a jelly sandwich. Denise explained that she really was not supposed to eat foods at other people's homes, including her grandmother's, but her grandmother assured her that this food was safe. Unfortunately, Denise had an allergic reaction. Denise's grandmother had previously made peanut butter and jelly sandwiches for her other grandchildren. She had accidentally used the same knife that was used for the peanut butter in the jelly jar, and so there was peanut butter mixed into the jelly jar. Denise's reaction was treated promptly. Denise's mother reviewed with Denise what had happened and why it was important that she only take food from individuals whom her mother indicated knew how to provide a safe meal for her.

Denise's grandmother was upset, but she wanted to learn how to provide safe foods for Denise. She discussed with her daughter how she could do so. Thanksgiving was upcoming, and Denise's grandmother wanted to be able to provide a safe Thanksgiving dinner for Denise and the entire family.

Because Denise was getting older and was going to be on her own more and also because her grandmother was so interested in learning about food allergy and providing a safe meal, it was decided that Thanksgiving would be a good opportunity for success. Denise's mother showed Denise's grandmother how to read labels and how to avoid cross-contact of foods. Denise's mother was confident Denise's grandmother had learned to make a safe meal.

Although no one is as likely as a parent or guardian to be educated and vigilant about safe meal preparation for their child, it is usually possible to achieve a comfort level with close friends and relatives as long as you know that they are well trained on how to provide a safe meal. Of course, this can be extended to restaurants, schools, camp cafeterias, or any location where someone may be preparing foods for your child. The level of education may depend on the foods your child avoids because it may be easier to prepare safe meals if there are fewer foods involved. To reduce stress at family gatherings, many families will bring foods prepared at home that can be served without concern. It may be possible to coordinate ahead of time the types of foods brought for your allergic child so that they essentially match the types of foods that the rest of the family would be eating for Thanksgiving or other holiday gatherings.

Emphasize to your child not to accept foods from individuals who have not been "approved" as able to provide a safe meal. Families will usually determine, on a case-by-case basis, their comfort level with particular individuals providing foods for their child. Sometimes relatives are offended if it is implied that they may not be able to provide a safe meal. I suggest that the adults involved meet with the family member separately to discuss the specifics of providing a safe meal. In regard to young food-allergic children who are not able to monitor themselves, large family gatherings where food is often spread out in many locations represents an increased risk because the young child may grab an allergenic food. Particular care must be taken to prevent accidental exposures in this setting by increasing direct supervision or moving food far from reach.

Friends, Play Dates, and Parties

Seven-year-old Lisa, who has milk, egg, peanut, and tree nut allergies, has enjoyed numerous play dates with her friends. However, friends always came to her home. Lisa's mother and father felt that it may not be safe for her to have play dates at her friends' homes because there may be risks and stress associated with snacks or foods eaten at these homes. They were also concerned about trying to instruct the friend's parents about epinephrine and emergency action plans for treating anaphylaxis. However, Lisa had been begging her parents to let her go to other children's homes for play dates. Lisa promised that she would not eat any foods at her friends' homes. Although her parents had considered perhaps letting her go on play dates without her medications, they were concerned that this would set a bad precedent and also was potentially unsafe, in the event Lisa were to have a reaction.

Lisa's family had good reason to be concerned. However, Lisa understood her allergies and how to control her diet. It seemed that Lisa would not intentionally eat food she was allergic to. I agreed with her parents that if Lisa went on a play date to the home of another child, she should bring her emergency medications, and the hosting family should be educated about her allergies. Approaching a family who has not dealt with food allergies or anaphylaxis could be a challenge. Introducing a family to new concepts about allergic reactions and medications used for treatment could be overwhelming and frightening. Some families may resist. I suggested that the family take an incremental approach to letting go, with the aim of allowing Lisa to play at other children's homes. Play dates were an important goal for her socialization and could likely be done with little risk.

We created a plan. Lisa's family would discuss her allergies with the adults at the friend's home. Lisa's parents explained that a food-allergic reaction was unlikely to occur because Lisa would not be eating any problematic foods while she was at their home. The family would not give Lisa any snacks. Lisa would bring her own food from home. As long as Lisa did not eat the foods prepared at her friend's home and did not participate in any food-related craft projects, an allergic reaction would be unlikely.

Her family also explained that Lisa typically at all times carries with her a written emergency action plan, epinephrine, and antihistamines in the event of an allergic reaction. Lisa had been trained how to report any symptoms to an adult and also how to use her medications, but her family also expressed concern that if Lisa were to have an allergic reaction, she might need an adult to help her to administer the medications and also to call 911. While Lisa's parents empathized with the host family that this could be a scary notion, it was actually quite simple to carry out the allergy action plan, and ultimately, very unlikely that it would be needed.

To reduce the possible stress involved, Lisa's mother asked to stay during the first play date. During the first play date, Lisa brought a snack and the two children ate their snack at the kitchen table. Of course, Lisa knew that there was no food sharing. Although Lisa's family did not feel that it was necessary for her friend to avoid milk, egg, peanut, or tree nut in her own diet during the visit, her friend volunteered to have a lunch and snack that did not contain these particular foods so that she could be more like Lisa during her snack time. During the play date, Lisa's mother showed her friend's mother how to administer the injectable epinephrine and Benadryl and reviewed the written emergency plan and contact numbers. The family's fears were allayed. At the second play date, Lisa's mother stayed for a shorter time. On the third play date, Lisa's mother did not stay. Lisa's parents successfully approached several other parents and soon Lisa was having play dates at the homes of other friends.

Children participate in many social activities with friends and families such as birthday parties and other celebrations. A little preparation can go a long way in these circumstances. I would usually not expect a friend's family to provide an allergen-free meal. It is usually simpler to prepare foods at home for your child with food allergies and bring these to the party. Find out the party menu ahead of time and consider making or buying a non-allergenic version of those dishes. Of course, you won't be able to do this every time. For younger children, it may be less stressful to try to stay at the party to supervise. But if there are close friends who understand about food allergy and have been trained about your child's emergency action plan, or if your child is older and capable, then it may be possible to approach birthday parties or other social activities with less trepidation and leave your child during the activity.

Often social activities with friends are food-centric. Families may have an ice cream sundae birthday party or some type of science party where crafts are made with foods. Always discuss with families what activities are planned. It may be difficult to expect a safe environment for your child at these parties. Explain to parents ahead of time the circumstances of your food-allergic child and your concerns about foods your child may encounter. Either excuse your child from the party or perhaps find an alternative way for your child to participate. Alternative activities that do not involve food may be possible.

One food-related activity that is a typical concern for children with food allergy is Halloween trick-or-treating. Although your child may not be able to ingest most, or perhaps any, of the candies they receive during trick-or-treating, this does not necessarily mean that your child cannot participate in the social activities of this type of holiday. You can make a deal ahead of time to have your child exchange with you the candy he cannot have for books, toys, safe snacks, or a movie. Before allowing your child to eat Halloween candy, read any labels on the wrapper. Unfortunately, many of the candies in individual servings will not have ingredient labels, so remove these.

A child with food allergies should still be able to participate in most social activities. With advanced preparation and understanding, it should be possible to have safe social experiences with your friends and relatives. In your own home, by following specific rules, families can have some of the allergenic foods available for other family members who are not allergic. However, sometimes it is easier for families to banish food allergens from their home. Whichever approach is chosen, keep all family members involved in these decisions.

21 ~ In Restaurants and while Traveling

Terry's family was hungry and looking forward to the first course of their restaurant meal. His parents had informed the waiter that 11-year-old Terry could not eat peanuts or tree nuts because he was allergic to these foods. Terry's salad was served with walnuts. The waiter apologized and removed the salad and served a new salad. After a few bites of lettuce, Terry complained of an itchy mouth. Apparently, the chef had only removed the top layer of the salad. However, small bits of walnut remained, which caused Terry's mouth to itch.

Eating in a restaurant poses a number of challenges for an individual with a food allergy. Most restaurants and various food service groups and organizations want to provide a safe meal for your child. I have lectured to restaurant staff and industry leaders about food allergy, and awareness among these groups about the need to provide safe meals is growing. However, obtaining a safe meal requires clear communication and cooperation from the person or family with the food allergy and the food handlers and preparers. My research group, in collaboration with the Food Allergy & Anaphylaxis Network, has performed studies identifying several pitfalls to ordering safe foods in restaurants. In this chapter, we will review ways to avoid these pitfalls and to obtain a safe meal in a restaurant during travel, and on vacation.

By serving a salad with nuts and by simply removing the nuts, the restaurant made two obvious errors in providing Terry's food. They definitely would benefit from education about food allergies. There are also several ways Terry's family could have reduced the risk of an error. Terry's family could have been more explicit with the restaurant to underscore that Terry would become ill even if he ingested trace amounts of nuts. Terry's family could have kept the original salad at the table and requested a new salad, thereby reducing the chance the restaurant would remove the nuts and re-serve the same salad. The family might also have considered discontinuing their meal at that restaurant, given the errors made.

Restaurant Meals

Emily is a 16-year-old girl with a fish allergy. She developed an allergic reaction in a restaurant after eating French fries. How did this happen? The fryer used to fry the potatoes had also been used to fry fish. This is an example of how cross-contact can contaminate a safe food. A different problem arose for Stephen. His parents selected a salad for him after reading ingredients on the menu. Stephen was allergic to peanuts, but no peanuts were listed for this salad. When the salad was served, Stephen's family confirmed with the waiter that the salad had been prepared without peanuts. However, Stephen had an allergic reaction to the salad. They discovered that the salad dressing contained peanut. How did this happen? Several errors occurred. First, the family relied on the menu to list all of the salad's ingredients. It's very risky to assume such a list would be accurate. Also, Stephen's parents did not inform the waiter that Stephen had a peanut allergy. The waiter may have assumed that Stephen just did not like peanuts. The waiter's response might have been different had the family stressed that Stephen had a potentially life-threatening allergy to peanuts and even a small amount could cause a reaction. Even if the restaurant staff personnel appear sensitive to food allergy issues, still ask the waiter or chef to identify the ingredients. A chef would have revealed that the dressing contained peanut sauce.

These are typical errors. We performed studies about food allergic reactions in restaurants for individuals who are peanut, nut, fish, or shellfish allergic. The types of errors that resulted in reactions were many but, thematically, could generally be traced to

poor communication, sometimes on the part of the family and other times on the part of the restaurant personnel;

cross-contact, meaning that pans, fryers, blenders, utensils, chopping boards, or cookware were contaminated by food containing the allergen;

simple human errors that perhaps could have been avoided if there were more awareness about food allergy.

Families dealing with food allergy must stress that their child has a *food allergy* and that even a small amount of the food can cause illness. "Chef cards" are helpful. These cards contain written summaries of the foods to which your child is allergic, with examples of foods and alternative words used for certain foods. The Food Allergy & Anaphylaxis Network (see Part 9) has examples of these cards that can be presented in a restaurant. The card may indicate exactly what your child is allergic to and also can serve as a starting point for conversations with the restaurant staff. While it may be helpful to speak with your waiter, the line of communication must really extend to the people who prepare the food. You would want to ensure that the individuals preparing the food understand how cross-contact may also be an issue. If a food is already partially prepared, then the individual who knows all the ingredients would need to be available to disclose whether the ingredients are safe for your child. Discuss your child's needs directly with the individual who prepared the food.

To ensure safety, know the chain of communication for everyone who is in contact with the food. For example, perhaps you have ordered plain steamed green beans for your child and the chef knows not to add any other ingredients. The steamed green beans are in a bowl and are perfectly safe for your child to ingest. However, if your child has milk allergies and the individual about to carry the bowl of string beans to your table thinks that they look rather dry and plain, he may add a little butter to make them look more appetizing. By the time the green beans reached the table, you would not know that a milk protein had been added. In some situations, it may not be possible to have adequate communication with the restaurant staff. Perhaps there are language barriers or it becomes clear that individuals are not "getting it." In these circumstances, I recommend families not to patronize that restaurant.

Another type of error that we discovered in our studies of restaurant allergies was cross-contact of allergens. A restaurant is a busy place, and it may be problematic to obtain food that has not touched an allergen. This does not mean that this is not an achievable goal, but there are some types of food selections that may be safer than others. Perhaps your child is milk allergic but tolerates beef. If the hamburger is grilled, it may come in contact with cheese or other foods prepared on the same grill. However, if the restaurant uses a clean pan and fries the hamburger in that pan alone, there would be likely no risk of cross-contact. This assumes, of course, that they are not preparing the meat ahead of time with added ingredients to which your child is allergic. Make sure the food preparers understand issues of cross-contact. Fryers, blenders, and other utensils that come in contact with food allergens should not come in contact with your child's food. Simple foods simply prepared (using clean utensils and cooking material) is a good rule of thumb. In some cases, fast-food establishments with regimented food-preparation procedures and dedicated fryers may pose fewer risks, but communication with the staff is still vital.

Depending on your child's specific food allergies, problems associated with cross-contact of allergens make some restaurants high risk. For individuals with peanut or nut allergy, bakeries are very difficult places to obtain safe foods because cross-contact is likely. Although it is possible to get a safe bakery product that does not contain peanuts or nuts, it would require a very careful discussion, extreme care, and advanced planning with the individuals in the bakery. Similarly, our studies have shown that Asian restaurants and ice cream parlors are very difficult locations to obtain safe meals for individuals with allergies to peanut or tree nut because of shared food-preparation items, such as woks. In an ice cream parlor, toppings can cross-contact with food that an individual with peanut or tree nut allergy may be ingesting. The ice cream scooper may not have been washed before your arrival and may have already spread peanuts or nuts into otherwise safe flavors when previously used. Sometimes the soft-serve ice cream is safer if you are not allergic to the ingredients in the ice cream. Salad bars and buffets present similar cross-contact problems. Customers may use the same serving tongs in different dishes, and food spills are frequent. Finally, if your child has a fish or shellfish allergy, then a seafood restaurant is probably a poor choice. Cross-contamination would be difficult to prevent.

What responsibility does a restaurant have for providing a safe meal? Restaurants do not want their patrons to have allergic reactions and strive to provide safe meals. However, restaurants also face certain limitations in what they can guarantee.

The Food Allergy & Anaphylaxis Network in partnership with the Food Allergy Initiative and the National Restaurant Association created restaurant programs that have been widely distributed. These programs teach restaurant personnel about food allergies, anaphylaxis, cross-contact in food preparation, and preparing safe meals for patrons with food allergies. In addition, the restaurant industry has attempted to increase awareness about food allergies and to provide educational materials to food service. Although it is likely that you will encounter more restaurant staff who are knowledgeable about food allergies, you must have specific conversations about your child's food allergies with food-preparation staff. If you are ever uncertain about the safety of a meal, do not eat it.

If your child experiences any symptoms while you are in the restaurant, you should follow your emergency action plan but also let the restaurant know of the problem. They should help you alert emergency services, such as calling 911. It may be helpful to also discuss with the restaurant what might have gone wrong so that you and the restaurant can avoid any pitfalls in the future. Write down all of the ingredients of the problem meal. I have advised my patients to keep the remainder of the meal in some cases, if it is unclear what they may have reacted to. It is always possible that some new food allergen has been introduced in a restaurant setting, and we would not want to assume that cross-contact of a previously diagnosed food allergen was the reason for the reaction when, perhaps, a new ingredient triggered the reaction.

If your child is allergic to food proteins that become airborne easily, it makes sense not to sit near the kitchen or exhaust area. Similarly, food cooked at the table may be a poor choice. Avoiding foods with sauces or prepared from buffets will also help to reduce the risk of cross-contamination. If your child has multiple food allergies and it is not possible to easily obtain a safe meal, then bring similar but safe foods to the restaurant for your child to eat along with the rest of the family. Explaining the situation to the restaurant will likely result in a pleasant experience.

A safe meal in a restaurant is possible if the right preparation and the right questions are asked. Carry written materials that you can show your server and chef. You want to work with the restaurant personnel to ensure a direct line of communication during all stages of food preparation. When the food is served, review with the waiter or chef that the meal was prepared safely. As your child gets older, you should involve them in these discussions so that they will feel comfortable ordering safe foods.

Travel

Judy's family was embarking on a trip to France. Judy is an 8-year-old with milk, egg, peanut, and tree nut allergy. She had not traveled outside of the country before and had never been on an airplane. The family had a list of questions about how they were going to be able to travel safely and also obtain safe meals for Judy. I explained to the family that we had quite a few things to discuss and quite a bit of preparation before their trip.

Judy had an emergency action plan, and typically carried self-injectable epinephrine and antihistamines. Because the family was going to be on a long plane trip, they wondered whether they should take extra epinephrine autoinjectors. An injection of epinephrine would perhaps be effective for five to twenty minutes, and usually only one dose is needed for an allergic reaction. Carrying two doses is recommended in case a second is needed; more than two doses is usually not needed. If an individual needs more than two or three doses of self-injectable epinephrine, they probably are quite ill and could benefit from additional therapies, such as intravenous fluids, available in an emergency room. Many families feel more comfortable carrying more than two doses of epinephrine when they travel, and I generally advise them to do so. For individuals whose travels take them to remote locations without medical facilities, I might advise that they carry additional medications, including oral steroids, in the event they could not receive additional medical help. For children with asthma, it is important to have the asthma medications available as well, even if asthma were in remission around the time of the trip. I reminded Judy's family to check expiration dates on the medications and to ensure they had the prescription and over-the-counter medications they needed before leaving for their trip.

Because of stricter airport security, families are concerned about carrying self-injectable epinephrine. I travel frequently for lectures and meetings, and I always carry two self-injectors of epinephrine. I have never been stopped nor prevented from boarding an airplane because of these injectors, and I have only been questioned once about carrying them. I carry a prescription with me to explain that the emergency medication is for an allergic reaction. Although it does not seem to be very common for individuals to be stopped for carrying the medication, it is possible. Therefore, I advise traveling families, like Judy's, to carry a signed note from a physician explaining the purpose of the medication. In addition, keep the pharmacy label on the medication.

What about airplane food? Although it may be possible to obtain an allergy-safe meal in an airplane, it is always safer to prepare food at home for your child to eat during the flight. Airline staff may question you about carrying on more than a small amount of food, which may be needed for long trips. Again, a note from your child's doctor may be useful.

Judy was allergic to peanuts and the family was concerned about peanuts being served on the airplane. In studies that we have performed regarding allergic reactions on airplanes, the most common cause of a peanut reaction on an airplane was eating them. Sometimes a young child found leftover peanuts in the seat or seat pockets and ate them. To avoid this problem, check the seating area for leftover food and peanut packages. Wipe off tray tables or seats to avoid casual exposure. I am not aware of reports of reactions to airborne foods on airplanes, aside from reports of possible reactions to peanut. In our studies, an allergic reaction from peanuts served on airplanes is rare, but when it has occurred, most reactions have been relatively mild and similar to reactions for individuals who, for example, are allergic to cats or dogs and are exposed to these animal danders. Reactions might include itchy eyes and sneezing, or for someone with a predilection toward asthma, possibly wheezing. Reactions in airplanes have been attributed to airborne exposure to peanut when large numbers of passengers open their packages of dry-roasted peanut at the same time. While there have been a few reports of more severe allergic reactions to peanuts on airplanes through air contact, these have been uncommon and hard to verify. I would be more concerned about foods being cooked on the airplane, which occasionally occurs. However, some airlines offer peanut-free flights. A list of these airlines can be found online through the Food Allergy & Anaphylaxis Network (see Part 9). By flying earlier in the day, you can avoid the time when peanut snacks would be served. Although Judy's family would carry all of her medications with them, airplanes also stock medications for emergencies.

In France, all of the issues that arise in obtaining a safe meal at home and in restaurants would become pertinent. The family was thinking about these issues in advance, and I encouraged them to call ahead to discuss with the hotel staff what measures could be taken to obtain safe meals in the hotel. The rules governing allergen labeling may be different in foreign countries than in the United States. Obtaining safe meals in supermarkets and restaurants can be difficult if you do not speak the native language. However, you would want to be sure to try to order simple foods prepared with safe ingredients. Avoiding sauces and staying away from foods with new or uncertain ingredients is prudent. By making some telephone calls in advance to restaurants, you may be able to determine the likelihood of obtaining safe meals, especially where communication is easier. Some of my patients have had their chef cards translated into the native language of the country they're visiting. However, to obtain a truly safe meal, it would be necessary to be able to communicate effectively with the individual who was preparing the food to ensure that the necessary precautions and preparations have taken place. The Food Allergy & Anaphylaxis Network has resources on traveling in and obtaining safe foods in different countries. When traveling in foreign countries, keep medications, a written emergency action plan, and medical identification jewelry with you at all times.

Vacations

Planning a vacation for a family with food allergies requires additional preparation, but a little preparation can go a long way in ensuring a safe and relaxing vacation. As discussed previously for foreign travel, make sure that your medications are up to date, that the emergency action plan is in place, that you have additional medications for allergies or asthma on hand, and that medical identification information is available. Many families contending with food allergies prefer vacations where they can prepare their own meals, say, at a resort or in a hotel kitchenette. In this way, the family can take some meals in restaurants or through food service but also prepare food for their child or children with food allergies in a safe manner. Many larger resorts now have become food-allergy aware, and it is possible to call ahead to discuss restaurant meal preparations. Even so, when you arrive, apply the practices you would use at home to obtain safe restaurant meals. Remind staff of your child's food allergies at every meal.

As you travel, it is helpful to have in mind what you would do in the event of an allergic reaction. This may include knowing where hospitals are located or how much time it may take to get medical attention. The more remote the location of your vacation or activities, the more certain you must be that all foods are safe.

An ocean-liner cruise may be more difficult for a family with a food-allergic child to take. Although a doctor may be onboard, advanced medical care for a severe allergic reaction would be more difficult to acquire and unless you brought your own food, most meals would be prepared on a large-scale basis. If you take a cruise, discuss ahead of time with the individuals involved in meal preparation whether safe meals can be obtained for your child. This may depend on the specific foods your child is allergic to and also on the abilities of the individuals preparing the foods on the cruise liner.

Enjoying meals at restaurants, while traveling, or on vacation without the stress of worrying about a food-allergic reaction requires preparation. Advanced preparation includes understanding the pitfalls and surmounting them by having available written materials explaining the allergy, making sure that you have a direct line of communication with the individuals preparing the food, and ensuring that food personnel understand the food allergy and the issues of cross-contact. Avoid foods with sauces and multiple ingredients or foods served at buffets or locations where cross-contamination is likely. Planning ahead of time will ensure an enjoyable vacation or restaurant meal with your child.

22 ~ At School and Camp

I had the pleasure of working with other parents and a teacher at my child's nursery school. During the half-day program, the children took a break to eat a snack provided by a parent. The children ate their snack at the same tables used for crafts and games, in the same room where all activities took place. A small washroom was also attached to this classroom. Before snack time, their tables were cleared of crafts or toys and wiped clean. The children were brought into the washroom, washed and dried their hands, and came back to the clean tables where the snack was served. The children had to eat their snack at the table, and they were not allowed to carry the snacks around the room. When snack time was over, all of the foods were cleaned away by the teacher and me, the children cleaned up and washed their hands, and the day continued. As a parent, I spent a fun day with my child. As an allergist, it occurred to me that had there been a food-allergic child in this classroom, the procedures already in place would have been sufficient to ensure a safe environment for the child.

Preschoolers tend to lick fingers and toys. The preschool cleaned up before and after the meal, which would have reduced the risk that foods would be spread to toys. The children ate their meal at the table and did not carry snacks around the room, which further decreased the risk of foods left in areas where an allergic child might have accidentally eaten or touched them.

Leaving your food-allergic child in the care of others at school or in camp can provoke anxiety. In this chapter, we will discuss ways in which you can help to ensure a safe environment for your child in school and at camp. Many of the specific details and procedures needed to keep your child safe will vary depending on the age of your child and the specific circumstances in the school. However, by recognizing potential pitfalls and understanding ways to avoid them, a safe school environment for your child should be achievable.

Studies about Food Allergy in Schools

A modest number of research publications focus on food allergy in the school setting. Our research group has undertaken studies to determine some of the issues that arise in schools. Although there is rightly much concern about peanut or tree nut allergy in the schools, one study showed that milk was the most common trigger of food-allergic reactions in the schools, not surprisingly because milk is a more ubiquitous food than peanut. Even though a larger number of children in schools had a peanut allergy, it was the children with milk allergy who were at a higher risk for accidentally ingesting a milk product. About 15 percent of food-allergic reactions in schools are treated with epinephrine, and most of the allergic reactions are treated with antihistamines. About 60 percent of the reactions are limited to skin symptoms, such as hives, while about 30 percent of the reactions included wheezing. Only rarely were blood-circulation problems noted.

A study we conducted targeted peanut or tree nut allergic reactions in schools. The average age of the children at the time of the survey was 11 years old, and the average age at the time of the reactions described was 4 years old. This seemed to indicate that the younger children were more prone to the allergic reactions. Most reactions occurred in daycare or preschool settings rather than in elementary or higher grades. Sixty percent of the reported reactions occurred from eating peanuts or foods with peanuts in them. In the youngest children, 1 in 4 of these allergic reactions to peanuts or tree nuts represented the child's first allergic reaction. One in 4 of the reactions were reported from skin contact. These were typically reactions only with skin symptoms, but ingesting the food in addition to touching the food could not be excluded for most. The triggering items included craft projects using peanut butter, such as making peanut butter bird feeders and handling various items with peanut. In 16 percent of the reactions, the trigger was attributed to possible inhalation of the food, although skin contact or eating the food could not be excluded. Only a few of these reactions were considered to be severe, and in only a few of the episodes did an adult believe that no ingestion of the food had occurred. One child's reaction occurred a foot away from a peanut fondue. Two occurred while children were making peanut butter bird feeders, and one occurred when the child was sitting with fifteen other children who were eating peanut butter crackers. It could not be verified that the children did not eat peanuts during these episodes.

For children with a particular food allergy, craft or cooking projects using the food should be avoided. The younger the child, the more likely the child is to have a reaction when the food is within reach. Because 1 in 4 of the reactions in young children in childcare was attributed to their first ingestion of peanut or tree nuts, childcare providers should be trained about food allergies and not serve highly allergenic foods to children for the first time. Last, for children with food allergies, and even for foods other than peanut, care must be taken to reduce the risks of an ingestion. These studies were undertaken primarily in the late 1990s and reflected reactions that occurred in the 1990s before widespread knowledge of food allergy and before many schools had established programs to keep children with food allergies safe.

School Guidelines

Linda, a 5-year-old with peanut allergy, was about to begin a full-day kindergarten program. In June before the school year, her mother met with the principal and school nurse to review Linda's food allergies. Linda's mother had compiled a list of rules she wanted the school to follow. The rules included not only an emergency action plan identifying allergic symptoms and how to treat them but also specific rules limiting what other children in the class could eat in school. Her plan included several pages with advice on cleaning the classroom, cleaning the school, and washing hands. Several pages included training modules for teachers and the school nurse. Linda's parents indicated that if the rules and procedures were not followed carefully, Linda might experience a fatal allergic reaction. Linda's parents were seeking a guarantee that the school could follow these procedures and ensure a safe environment. The school principal and nurse were concerned that they would not likely be able to follow all of the procedures. Although they had many procedures in place for children with food allergies, they could not follow all of the suggestions that Linda's family had outlined, which disturbed Linda's parents.

Linda's family overwhelmed the school with the specifics of her care plan, and all sides saw potentially insurmountable obstacles. I recommend that families approach a school in advance, as Linda's parents had done. However, I suggest that families first determine what precautions the school has already implemented because most schools have experience with children with allergies. What policies and procedures does the school already offer to provide a safe environment for a child with food allergies? The general principle of a school plan is to reduce the chance that the child will ingest the food allergen and to have procedures that recognize and treat an allergic reaction appropriately and promptly. Specifics of the plan will depend on many factors and will vary from school to school, grade to grade, and child to child. Some states provide suggested guidelines to school systems. In addition, the National Association of Elementary School Principals, the American Food Service Association, the National Association of School Nurses, the National School Board Association, and the Food Allergy & Anaphylaxis Network have developed school guidelines for food allergies. These guidelines identify three primary areas of responsibilities:

Family's Responsibility

Notify the school of the child's allergies.

Work with the school team to develop a plan that accommodates the child's needs throughout the school, including in the classroom, in the cafeteria, in after-care programs, during school-sponsored activities, and on the school bus, as well as a Food Allergy Action Plan.

Provide written medical documentation, instructions, and medications as directed by a physician, using the Food Allergy Action Plan as a guide. Include a photo of the child.

Provide properly labeled medications and replace expired or expended medications.

Educate the child in the self-management of their food allergy, including the following:

- safe and unsafe foods
- strategies for avoiding exposure to unsafe foods
- symptoms of allergic reactions
- how and when to tell an adult they may be having an allergy-related problem
- how to read food labels (age appropriate)

Review policies and procedures with the school staff, the child's physician, and the child (if age appropriate) after a reaction has occurred.

Provide emergency contact information.

School's Responsibility

Know and follow applicable federal laws, including the Americans with Disabilities Act, Section 504, and any state laws or district policies that apply.

Review the health records submitted by parents and physicians.

Include food-allergic students in school activities. Students should not be excluded from school activities solely based on their food allergy.

Identify a core team of, but not limited to, school nurse, teacher, principal, school food service and nutrition manager/director, and counselor (if available) to work with parents and the student (age appropriate) to establish a prevention plan. Changes to the prevention plan to promote food allergy management should be made with core team participation.

Assure that all staff who interact with the student regularly understand food allergy, can recognize symptoms, know what to do in an emergency, and work with other school staff to eliminate the use of food allergens in the allergic student's meals, educational tools, arts and crafts projects, or incentives.

Practice the Food Allergy Action Plans before an allergic reaction occurs to ensure the efficiency/effectiveness of the plans.

Coordinate with the school nurse to be sure medications are appropriately stored and that an emergency kit is available that contains a physician's standing order for epinephrine. Some states permit medications to be kept in an easily accessible, secure location central to designated school personnel, not in locked cupboards or drawers. Students should be allowed to carry their own epinephrine (if age appropriate), if allowed by state or local regulations with approval from the students' physician or clinic, parents, and school nurse.

Designate school personnel who are properly trained to administer medications in accordance with the State Nursing and Good Samaritan Laws governing the administration of emergency medications.

Be prepared to handle a reaction and ensure that a staff member is available who is properly trained to administer medications during the school day regardless of time or location.

Review policies/prevention plan with the core team members, parents/guardians, student (age appropriate), and physician after a reaction has occurred.

Work with the district transportation administrator to assure that school bus driver training includes symptom awareness and what to do if a reaction occurs.

Recommend that all buses have communication devices in case of an emergency.

Enforce a "no eating" policy on school buses with exceptions made only to accommodate special needs under federal or similar laws, or school district policy.

Discuss appropriate management of food allergy with family.

Discuss field trips with the family of the food-allergic child to decide appropriate strategies for managing the food allergy.

Follow federal/state/district laws and regulations regarding sharing medical information about the student.

Take threats or harassment against an allergic child seriously.

Student's Responsibility

Must not trade food with others.

Must not eat anything that contains unknown ingredients or is known to contain any allergen.

Be proactive in the care and management of their food allergies and reactions based on their developmental level.

Notify an adult immediately if they eat something they believe may contain the food to which they are allergic.

These general guidelines are designed to help reduce a child's risk of an allergic reaction and if a reaction occurs to have the means to identify and treat an allergic reaction. In addition to these general guidelines, excellent resources from the Food Allergy & Anaphylaxis Network are available to help schools manage food allergies (see Part 9). Many specifics in these resources follow the recommendations of the various organizations responsible for the school guidelines. Even though these guidelines now exist, many concerns arise regarding the care of children in school settings. In the following section, we will consider some of the common concerns that arise in providing a safe school environment for children with food allergies. You are encouraged to discuss the specific issues for your child with your pediatrician, allergist, and school personnel. Unfortunately, the effectiveness of suggestions made by professional organizations has not been extensively evaluated.

Common Concerns

Understanding the Action Plan

A written action plan should include your child's name, picture, what your child is allergic to, symptoms of an allergic reaction, contact information, medication information, and procedures. In addition, medications such as self-injectable epinephrine and antihistamines must be available for your child. In our studies of food-allergic reactions in schools, we have identified several components of the action plan often associated with pitfalls and errors. Sometimes, confusion arose because it was not clear who was responsible for carrying out the action plan. Usually, a school nurse, if available, was designated to carry out an emergency plan and to identify others who would participate. A team approach is often needed to identify, report, and treat an allergic reaction. For example, schoolteachers, the principal, and a lunchroom supervisor should be educated to be able to identify an allergic reaction and should know what actions to take. Everyone should know and review their roles. Another point of confusion identified in our studies was the location of the emergency medications. Some schools prefer to keep the medication in the nurse's office or in the principal's office. In other circumstances, schools prefer to have the medication in a teacher's room or sometimes in several locations. Perhaps the most important point is that the medication is available in unlocked cabinets, earmarked for the child with food allergies, and everyone responsible for your child knows where to find medications and how and when to use them.

Confusion arises when specific responsibilities have not been assigned and reviewed. Although a child may be carrying her own medications, an adult should ultimately be responsible for administering, or helping to administer, the medications and also helping to decide when the medications are needed and judging the response to treatment. Knowing who is designated to help your child is important; however, ensuring that everyone knows the specifics of activating an emergency action plan is crucial. In other words, if the schoolteacher notices that your child is having a reaction, what will he do? Perhaps the procedure would be to bring your child directly to the school nurse, or perhaps the procedure would be to evaluate and treat the child without going to the school nurse. Who should evaluate and treat your child should be decided in advance. It would be most appropriate to have a school nurse perform the assessment if a school nurse is available, which would put a health professional in charge.

Because a reaction may proceed quickly, some believe notifying the school nurse would waste time or delay treatment. How prompt is prompt in treating an allergic reaction? The answer may affect how an action plan is carried out; unfortunately, there is no perfect answer. Fatalities associated with food allergies have typically occurred when treatment was significantly delayed, for example, more than twenty minutes from the onset of symptoms. Thus, it could be argued that spending a few minutes locating a healthcare professional, such as a school nurse, may be worthwhile for accurately evaluating the symptoms, deciding whether medications or which medications are needed, and judging responses to treatment. The time it takes to find the nurse could vary depending on the size of the school and the location of the nurse in relation to the child in need. Many schools have an intercom system that may facilitate locating the nurse. Nonetheless, a few moments of delay may be advantageous.

As discussed in Chapter 2, many symptoms may mimic anaphylaxis. For example, it is possible to confuse a sore throat with throat tightness, an asthmatic episode with an allergic reaction, or a mosquito bite with hives. In all of these circumstances, I could argue that a school principal, who is not a qualified healthcare professional, should treat such symptoms as possible anaphylaxis because the principal is not trained to know exactly what may cause these symptoms, and I might want the principal to err on the side of treatment. However, a school nurse may be able to make a more refined assessment and may identify another cause of the symptoms, which would not require anaphylaxis treatment. The delay in treatment during the time it takes to get your child to the nurse must be considered against the benefit of having the nurse, rather than another adult with no healthcare experience, evaluate your child. The best procedures for your child may need to be individualized, depending on your child's allergies, prior reactions, and specific circumstances in a given school.

Key points in the action plan must be considered and reviewed:

1. Designated persons must understand the exact technique for self-administered epinephrine.
2. Strongly consider having your child wear medical identification jewelry.
3. Ensure that appropriate contact numbers are available and that emergency services will be contacted before trying to reach the parents or others.
4. Ensure that medications are up to date and readily available.

5. Ensure that designated individuals who know about your child's food allergy understand how to recognize symptoms, know how to treat symptoms with medications, and follow the emergency action plan.

6. Ensure that provisions are in place to communicate these issues to substitute teachers.

The emergency action plan should be practiced like a fire drill. It may not be appropriate, for emotional reasons in some situations, to include your child in these drills, but it can be considered, especially for older children. Practice runs would include the individuals involved—including those who would contact the nurse, stay with your child, treat with medications, and dial 911. In addition, the trial run would ensure the medications are available and their use understood. Practicing not only prepares the participants but also helps identify and fix any problems in the plan.

Unsafe Activities

Julian is a 6-year-old boy with egg allergy who experienced swelling of the eyes while finger painting at school. The teacher had smoothed the finger paints with egg white, which caused Julian's reaction. When putting together plans for the school, it is important to identify the activities that may pose a special risk for individuals with food allergies. In craft projects, egg might be used in finger painting, peanut might be used to make peanut butter–covered bird feeders, and wheat might be used in modeling clay. School activities may include cooking projects, which may aerosolize the foods or result in significant skin contact leading to symptoms. Many of my patients' families describe activities where young children are requested to count foods such as nuts. With sensory games children may be blindfolded and asked to feel, taste, or sniff objects, sometimes foods, to determine what they may be. These games and crafts using foods pose undue dangers for children with food allergies and should be discouraged or substitutions with safe materials found. When you are reviewing an action plan with your school, you should ensure that they have a consciousness for these exposures and that your child's teacher and also arts and crafts teacher, rotating teachers, and substitutes know about these potential exposures and how to avoid them. Alternative foods might be selected and craft projects that do not include foods could be developed.

Exposures through Skin and Air

Concerns about allergic reactions from casual contact such as sniffing or touching are a source of anxiety because these are very difficult exposures to control. As reviewed in Chapter 2 on anaphylaxis, casual contact, meaning skin contact without ingestion, is unlikely to cause a severe allergic reaction. However, it is always possible that a larger exposure may cause a more significant reaction, or a small exposure to certain areas of the body, even without ingestion, may cause reactions that may appear dramatic. For example, getting a food allergen into the eye can cause significant eyelid swelling. To aerosolize food, it is usually necessary to cook it or have a large amount of exposure. Nonetheless, there are concerns about the possibility of a young child touching a food (then touching her mouth) or licking objects in the classroom that are contaminated with food. This concern has led to the consideration of banning particular foods and undertaking measures to reduce an exposure by washing hands and by cleaning various classroom objects.

While taking measures to reduce casual contact exposure has been part of plans to help to keep food-allergic children safe, it has also been a source of anxiety and frustration for several reasons. First, trying to eliminate completely the potential for an exposure by skin contact may be difficult to achieve in a practical sense. Families with food-allergic children with these concerns wonder whether other individuals entering the school have carried the food on their person, and individuals who are not allergic may feel that burdens are being placed on them with unclear benefits for the allergic child. Schools have concerns about whether they can banish a particular targeted allergen and may feel unable to control completely all of the circumstances in the school building. Families wonder whether hand washing will really eliminate the allergen. When bans are instituted, questions arise about whether these restrictions really keep food out of the building. Even among families with food-allergic children, there are sometimes conflicts regarding banning one particular food over another, for example, peanuts rather than milk or eggs.

Although these stressful issues and concerns have no perfect answers, it is sometimes helpful to consider the degree of risk associated with these exposures and what efforts may be reasonable in a variety of settings. For example, it may be more significant to clean the hands of young children who are more prone to licking their fingers. In one study that performed wipe sampling of various surfaces in several schools, most surfaces with no apparent peanut protein had none detectable during the random sampling.

When peanut was detectable, it was in an amount that would not be expected to cause a reaction even if a child, for example, had licked the entire surface. Obviously, the situation would be different if a food was actually noticeable on the surface. For example, if a child with milk allergy was eating at a table, milk spilled on the tabletop, spread to the child's food, and the allergic child ate the food, there would be a great concern. If a young child was prone to licking surfaces and a similar situation arose, that would be troubling too. Thus, the same exposure can result in different risks depending on the age and abilities of the child.

I am not aware of any studies showing that an environmental exposure to food allergens is different than an environmental exposure to typical airborne allergens. For example, a bit of milk protein on playground equipment should not pose more of a danger than pollen on that equipment, unless the child licked the equipment. During pollen season, it is possible to see a sheen of yellow or green on outdoor surfaces, such as the car hood. Playground equipment, such as monkey bars, may be coated with this allergen. Children with pollen allergies playing on the equipment might rub their eyes with pollen-contaminated fingers and develop itchy and swollen eyelids but usually not much more than that. While parents may be concerned that a child would contaminate monkey bars with a food such as milk, it is more likely that the monkey bars would be covered with pollen. For the pollen-allergic child, I recommend that parents encourage them not to touch their eyes or mouth and to wash their hands and clean themselves when they are done. The same advice applies to the family of a milk-allergic child concerned about playground equipment that may have milk contamination that is not visible. The milk-reaction risk should be extremely low considering that only a trace amount, if any, would remain on the equipment. Certainly, if a child is old enough to understand what she's allergic to, she'll avoid touching that food if it's stuck on playground equipment or wash her hands if she got them dirty.

In regard to hand cleaning, in one study, adults purposely placed a teaspoon of peanut butter on their hands and then cleaned them. Washing with soap and running water or using commercial wet wipes efficiently removed peanut from their hands; however, water alone or a hand sanitizer did not removed the peanut. No studies of children cleaning food proteins from their hands have been conducted. One could argue for hand cleaning based on good hygiene, but it is unclear to what extent hand cleaning can protect children from contact with food allergens. Hand washing may be an issue for preschool-age children because licking toys or tables may be more likely.

Each school must consider various options to reduce exposure to food allergens. Some schools perform schoolwide bans of certain food proteins. Some schools will ban particular foods for certain classrooms where meals are eaten in the classroom. Many schools have taken to having peanut-free or allergy-free tables where individuals who are not eating the foods to which the child is allergic sit with the child with food allergies. For example, they may be having juice instead of milk. In my experience, as children progress to higher grades, they often no longer want to sit at these tables and are willing to follow strict no-food-sharing rules. In addition, for older children, concerns about casual skin exposures leading to licking/oral ingestion are minor compared with food sharing or taking unsafe food. As the guidelines indicate, it is vital for food-allergic children to know that they cannot share foods, utensils, straws, or drinking cups with other children.

If a belligerent child in a classroom of any age were trying to hurt an allergic child by exposing him to a food, the bullying child would need to be instructed about the seriousness of his actions and action would need to be taken to prevent future bullying.

Meals in School

I usually advise families to provide their child's food for the school day. Parents could provide nonperishable snacks and store them at the school so that substitutions are available for parties and celebrations. However, some schools with cafeteria service are willing and able to provide safe meals for a food-allergic child. It is still important to have a careful conversation with the school personnel to be clear that they are trained in label reading and safe food preparation to avoid cross-contamination with allergenic foods.

The School Bus

The school bus is often a particular point of anxiety because the bus driver is not a healthcare professional, and no school nurse is available to evaluate a reaction. However, the bus driver should be trained to recognize food allergies and to know when such an emergency is occurring so that she can call 911. The school bus driver should also be aware of the location of local hospitals, although it may be more efficient to call 911 if an allergic reaction occurred.

The primary goal of the bus ride is to avoid allergic reactions. Therefore, the child should not eat while on the school bus. If your child is not eating anything on the school bus, then it is unlikely that he would have a reaction on the school bus, unless he ate something right before boarding. On the way to school, presumably, a safe meal would have been eaten at home. On the way home, if your child has not eaten for an hour or so before boarding the bus, it is unlikely that a food-allergic reaction would occur so long after the last meal, particularly a safe meal. If a reaction is detected before your child boards the bus, then he should not be put on the school bus. In fact, one of the sources of error that we discovered in our research studies was that a child who was having an allergic reaction was rushed onto the bus with the idea that he would go home for his family to evaluate him rather than keeping him at the school and following his action plan. If there is some concern that your child may be eating at school soon before getting on a bus, it may be sensible to have your child quickly checked before sending them off on the bus. Some families feel more comfortable having their child sit at the front of the bus under the bus driver's watchful eye.

School Trips

Field trips require special consideration because healthcare personnel or individuals who are usually designated to care for your child in the event of an allergic reaction may not be on the trip. There must be adults on the trip who are designated to care for your child in the event of an emergency. All of the action plans and emergency medications must be on hand and reviewed before the trip. It is unlikely that acquiring a safe meal would be an easy undertaking for most school trips. Therefore, provide a safe meal for your child to reduce the risk of a reaction. Certain trips are not good choices for children with a food allergy. For example, it may not be fair or reasonable to take a trip to food manufacturing factories or a trip that includes projects using foods or cooking. Extended trips would require the same care that was discussed in Chapter 21 regarding vacations.

Carrying Epinephrine

Many states allow children to carry emergency medications, such as asthma medications and self-injectable epinephrine. What age is appropriate to allow a child to carry the medications, and what age is appropriate to allow a child to decide on self-administration of medications? Maturity more so than age will determine when a child is ready for these responsibilities. Certain children may not be responsible for carrying their medications around because they may play with the medications and potentially injure themselves or another child. Or if the child with the allergy is trustworthy to safely carry the medication, some of the children around him may be irresponsible and may tamper with the medication, exposing themselves and others to injury. A child's ability to understand and treat his illness will determine whether he can carry the medication and be trusted to use it appropriately. (Even some adults are reluctant to self-medicate.) For these reasons, a designated adult should always be available to administer medications. However, if a child is deemed by his school, his family, and his physician to be responsible to carry medications safely and to self-administer, then allow it. Sometimes children forget or lose their medications, so have backup medications at home and in unlocked locations within the school building.

Guidelines for carrying and using medications in school has been summarized by various national professional organizations (a copy of the full report is available through the Web site of the American Academy of Pediatrics; see Part 9, Food Allergy Resources). These organizations recognize that eventually a student should understand, carry, and administer her own medication. However, they also recognize that doing so within a school setting should be weighed against available school resources. If a school has adequate resources and adheres to policies that promote safe and appropriate administration of lifesaving medications by school personnel, there could be less relative benefit, especially for less mature students, to carry and self-administer medication. In contrast, if resources were inadequate, there would be a stronger reason to have a student carry and self-administer. Some of the factors of relevance in deciding to allow carrying and self-administration include the following:

STUDENT

- desire to carry and self-administer epinephrine
- appropriate age, maturity, or developmental level
- ability to identify signs and symptoms of anaphylaxis
- knowledge of proper medication use in response to signs/symptoms
- ability to use correct technique in administering epinephrine
- knowledge about medication side effects and what to report
- willingness to comply with school's rules about use of medicine at school, for example:

    keeping the autoinjector of epinephrine with him/her at all times

    notifying a responsible adult (e.g., teacher, nurse, coach, playground assistant) *immediately* when autoinjectable epinephrine is used

    not sharing medication with other students or leaving it unattended not using autoinjectable epinephrine for any other use than what is intended

PARENT OR GUARDIAN

- desire for the student to self-carry and self-administer
- awareness of school medication policies and parental responsibilities
- commitment to making sure the student has the needed medication with them, medications are refilled when needed, backup medications are provided, and medication use at school is monitored through collaborative effort between the parent/guardian and the school team

504 Plans

Nowadays it seems that most schools are familiar with the management of children with food allergies, even multiple food allergies. Typically, you will find that your school has a variety of measures in place that will meet the needs of your child. However, sometimes situations arise in which families have difficulty working with the school. Some families turn to laws that may help them achieve goals for a safe school experience. The Americans with Disabilities Act Title III indicates that "no individual shall be discriminated against on the basis of disability, and to the full and equal enjoyment of the goods and services of any public accommodation." In addition, the Rehabilitation Act of 1973 Section 504, Public Law 93-112, discusses the prohibition of discrimination in education for any type of handicap. This law applies to programs and institutions that receive federal funds. The Section 504 plan was initially developed for children with educational disabilities, such as learning disabilities, blindness, or deafness, to ensure that these children received the services they need for a proper education.

This same law has been applied to help children with diabetes, seizures, or food allergies. The Section 504 Plan, in regard to food allergies, could be set up to require the school to have a plan that makes it safe for your child to attend the school and learn effectively. It would ensure an emergency plan is in place and that substitutions are identified so that your child can participate in activities with the other children. Most of my patients do not develop 504 plans because they are able to work with the administration and the school nurse to accommodate the child's needs. However, if you are having trouble with a school providing a safe environment and the school receives federal funds, a 504 plan can help you achieve the needed goals.

Comprehensive programs available through the Food Allergy & Anaphylaxis Network describe many ways that schools can help to create a safe environment for children with food allergies. You should further discuss the nuances of your particular plan with school personnel and with your physician. Never forget that your child is an important component of this plan. Your child is responsible for not trading food with others, for understanding the use of their medications, and for letting an adult know immediately of any allergic reaction.

Camp

Most concerns regarding school safety apply to camps. However, certain problematic circumstances may arise in summer camp. Teenagers are often responsible for direct supervision of your child and may not understand allergies. You want to ensure that persons are responsible and well educated about food allergies, including the teenagers who may be supervising your child as well as the camp nurse and/or supervising adults. You may need to review the specifics of the care plan for your child frequently, including all of the procedures associated with meals or snacks and also what to do in the event of an allergic reaction. Because a camp may be spread out geographically, a child may need to carry his emergency medications on his person or have them carried by a counselor. This may also be an issue when campers are hiking. Because many camp activities include foods and interactions with individuals aside from those specifically assigned to your child, for example, a nature specialist or arts and crafts specialist, all of these individuals should be educated about your child's food allergy and that the foods to which your child is allergic should not be included in any craft projects. If additional camp personnel are likely to be responsible for your child at some point, they must also be educated about your child's food allergies.

All of the same diligence that applies to meals at school applies to meals eaten at camp. However, it is generally not practical to provide meals for your food-allergic child if they are attending an overnight camp. Therefore, it would be important that those providing the meals for your child know the details of safe meal preparation.

Interview the individuals involved in caring for your child at overnight camp. In particular, you will want to interview medical and food preparation staff, emphasizing many of the same issues discussed earlier for managing food allergies in schools. If your child's camp is far from your home, you may also wish to ensure that a healthcare facility is close to the camp and perhaps alert a pediatrician, an allergist, and the hospital of your child's proximity. Many of the overnight camps have a designated camp physician who can review with you and with your child's usual pediatrician and allergist the specific issues. The specific decisions about which types of camps and what procedures to undertake in the camp will, of course, need to be individualized depending on your child, your child's age, specific food allergies, severity of the food allergy, and the ability of the camp to provide safe food, identify an allergic reaction, and provide care.

Successful food-allergy management plans require a coordinated and cooperative effort among a team of individuals, including yourself, your child, school, or camp personnel, particularly the nurse and additional faculty such as teachers, principals, coaches, counselors, food service, and bus drivers. Your allergist and pediatrician should be able to help guide you for some of your child's needs, but because the school or camp is individualized, the specific procedures that work best for your child and your school often need to be decided on by school or camp health professionals and administrators. Excellent programs for managing food allergy in schools, camps, and childcare are available from the Food Allergy & Anaphylaxis Network (Part 9). Ensuring that a plan is in place well ahead of the summer, before the school season begins, and many months in advance of the camp stay, with a review of the procedures at the beginning of the school or camp season, will best ensure the safety of your child.

PART 5

FOOD ALLERGY AT DIFFERENT AGES AND STAGES

A great joy in raising a child is watching your child grow and develop. From infancy, when your baby is completely dependent on you for everything, to the toddler years, when exploration takes precedence and your 2-year-old learns how to manipulate the world around them, you included. The preschool years are a time of learning more about the world and exercising independence while socializing. Through the early school-age years, your child is more independent, as she becomes her own person. In the teen and young adult years, your child is finding her way and probably finding trouble in the process. For children with food allergies, each childhood stage has specific challenges you and your child will face together.

In Part 5, I explore some of the most common age-specific issues that arise for children and families with food allergies. Particular points of focus include how to approach the diet and how to look for resolution of food allergies, or, in some cases, the development of new food allergies or other allergic problems. I consider how your child will take on, with your guidance, increasing responsibilities for protecting herself in regard to food allergies, and making successful transitions as she gets older, is more independent, and faces new challenges. Of course, every child is different, and no single recipe for success exists, but as is the case for all aspects of caring for your child with food allergies, understanding some of the challenges that may arise will help you to meet them successfully.

23 ~ Infants and Toddlers

Seven-month-old Michelle had been breast-fed since birth and had started on several solid foods. Michelle had been doing well, but when she was fed yogurt, her first cow's milk product, she developed hives. An allergy evaluation revealed positive tests for milk and egg. Michelle's mother had been eating a variety of typically allergenic foods, such as egg, milk, peanuts, nuts, and fish. She had many questions about how her diet might affect Michelle.

Breast-Feeding

Breast-feeding is the recommended form of infant nutrition. Babies should be exclusively breast-fed for the first four to six months. For infants with food allergies, two issues arise involving the nursing mother's diet. First, does the nursing mother's diet influence the development of allergy in an infant? This topic will be examined in Chapter 29. Second, could what Michelle's mother ingests cause an allergic reaction in Michelle? What a nursing mother ingests may be passed into her breast milk. The amount of protein passed from mother to child is extremely low in comparison to what would be the case if the infant ingested the food directly. In addition, how much protein a mother may pass to her breast milk and the time period over which it is present vary.

Research shows that allergenic proteins, such as milk, egg, or peanut, can make their way into the mother's breast milk. In a study of twenty-three women who ate peanut on purpose, the protein was detectable in the breast milk of half of the mothers. In those mothers, detectable peanut protein in their breast milk peaked about one hour after they had eaten it. After four hours of expressing breast milk samples hourly, all but 2 of 11 women still had detectable peanut protein in their breast milk.

If food proteins can enter the breast milk, should a mother whose child is allergic to the particular foods avoid them? This is not easy to answer. For Michelle, until she ingested cow's milk protein directly in the form of yogurt, there was no indication her mother's breast milk was a problem, even though her mother was on an unrestricted diet that included cow's milk. Allergic reactions from proteins ingested by a nursing mother are apparent in some infants. For example, some infants may have bloody stools, which are attributed to maternal ingestion of cow's milk protein. Avoiding cow's milk protein resolves the problem. Severe eczema symptoms, such as skin rash, in infants may dissipate when mothers discontinue, or significantly reduce, the ingestion of allergenic foods. Rare reports recount infants' sudden or severe allergic reactions from breast-feeding following the maternal ingestion of a food to which the infant is allergic.

For Michelle, who was growing well, having no stomach problems, and no rashes, it did not seem necessary for her mother to remove allergenic foods from her own diet while breast-feeding. Whether to remove those foods is also a personal decision you should discuss with your doctor. One could raise theoretical concerns that continued ingestion could "increase" the allergy or that eventually a reaction might occur, but no studies confirm that theory, and no current evidence existed of a problem for Michelle. If Michelle had skin rashes, gastrointestinal problems, or growth issues, her mother would have been advised to avoid the potential allergens. Michelle's mother decided to keep egg and milk in her diet in the amount she had previously consumed.

Infant Formula

Unlike Michelle, Kayla, a 5-month-old who was diagnosed with multiple food allergies, was not originally doing well as she breast-fed. While her mother was breast-feeding in the early months, Kayla was experiencing severe atopic dermatitis requiring numerous therapies. Kayla's mother excluded all of the major food allergens from her own diet, and a dietitian helped her to maintain a nutritious diet. Kayla's skin improved, although problems persisted. Kayla's mother wanted to start her on formula. Several hypoallergenic formulas are on the market for children with milk allergy.

The typical infant formula is a cow's milk protein–based formula that has been modified in ways to provide adequate nutrition for infants. The protein in typical cow's milk–based formula is unmodified. Recall from Chapter 1 that proteins are chains of molecules called amino acids; we can imagine each amino acid to be like a bead on a baby's bracelet. The regular cow's milk infant formula would, therefore, have proteins that spell out the word "C-O-W'-S-M-I-L-K-P-R-O-T-E-I-N." There are also formulas on the market called *partial hydrolysates.* In these formulas, the milk protein is broken into smaller pieces that may have less of an allergic effect. In this case, imagine the baby's bracelet chopped into smaller pieces floating around such as C-O-W, M-I-L-K, W-S-M-I, and so on. Although this formula is less allergic, the immune systems of Kayla or Michelle are likely to identify these pieces of cow's milk protein, and it is likely that Michelle or Kayla would have an allergic reaction from this formula. An extensive hydrolysate is a formula based on cow's milk protein. With these formulas, the baby's bracelet has been chopped into much smaller pieces. Now we have floating around M-I, L-K, P-R-O, and so on. Most infants' immune systems, even though they have already mounted a response against cow's milk protein, will not detect the residual small pieces of cow's milk protein in these formulas. These formulas must be fed to approximately thirty cow's milk–allergic infants who must all tolerate the formula in order to declare it "hypoallergenic" for children with cow's milk allergy. This testing does not exclude the possibility that some children may react to this formula. In some studies, it has been found that almost 2 percent of cow's milk–allergic children may still have an allergic response to this formula. Presumably, these infants' immune systems are able to recognize that these small chains, or pieces, of cow's milk protein are present.

An amino acid–based formula is not derived from cow's milk protein or other animal proteins but rather is a formulation of the separate amino acids, or baby's bracelet beads in our example. These formulas are more expensive and not very tasty but are unlikely to cause an allergic response for any infants. The taste declines as you move from cow's milk–based formula to the partially hydrolyzed to the extensively hydrolyzed, and then finally to the amino acid–based formulas.

Soy formulas are a poor choice for an allergy-prone infant because soy is one of the common food allergens for infants. Discuss with your pediatrician and allergist whether soy formula is an option, particularly if your child is already drinking it with no adverse effects. Both Kayla and Michelle were able to tolerate an extensively hydrolyzed milk-based formula. Because of the significant change in taste, Michelle's and Kayla's mothers introduced the formula by gradually adding the extensive hydrolysate formula to their expressed breast milk.

New Allergies

The *allergic march,* or *atopic march,* are terms used to describe the unfortunate fact that many infants with food allergies or atopic dermatitis later develop other allergic problems, such as asthma or hay fever. An infant may outgrow some allergies or develop new ones. Therefore, I caution parents of children such as Michelle or Kayla to watch carefully for symptoms of new allergies. Because of the asthma risk, watch for chronic cough or any signs of disturbed breathing, such as fast breathing or retractions (when the chest pulls in as the child breathes). These may be signs of asthma and would require medical attention. Although Michelle and Kayla had not experienced these problems, I told them what to look for and to call their pediatrician or me should these symptoms occur.

In the first year of life, new food allergies may still be developing or, less commonly, may be resolving. The target of problems always centers on the major food allergens: milk, eggs, wheat, soy, peanuts, tree nuts, and seafood. An allergic response can result from any food; however, these are the major allergenic foods. Once it is established that an infant has food allergies, avoid introducing more significant food allergens until further testing and evaluation has been undertaken. This leaves, of course, plenty of foods that could be tried during the first year. Cooked versions of fruits and vegetables and some of the grains are good choices in these early months. Of course, read labels to ensure that major allergens are not present. For example, it is highly unlikely that an infant would react to broccoli, but whenever I receive a call that one of my patients has, I ask the family to check the label, and sure enough, butter has been added to the jar of baby food. The reaction was actually caused by the milk rather than the broccoli.

Consult with your pediatrician and allergist to select the best food choices for your infant. To reduce risk start with orange fruits and vegetables in cooked form, including sweet potato, squash, and carrot. Apple, peach, or plum in jars are usually well tolerated; then introduce oat, rice, and corn, followed by wheat, which is typically more allergenic. It may be avoided or delayed in a child with milk allergy. The specific food choices may vary depending on your infant's prior reactions and types of allergic problems. For example, oat and rice may be delayed longer in an infant who has enterocolitis syndrome (see Chapter 4).

Toddlers

Ira is a 20-month-old who seems to have entered the "terrible twos" a bit early. He loves to explore and topple things over. Look away for a few seconds and Ira will find his way into the garbage can. If he does not get his way, he screams and cries until he does. These typical challenges were compounded because of Ira's multiple food allergies. I would be addressing a variety of issues with Ira's family to keep him safe during his toddler years.

Independence, Safety, and Socializing

Ira is too young to understand the dangers of grabbing the wrong food or rummaging through the garbage. Ira's natural curiosity and independence presented specific challenges that had to be addressed at home and elsewhere. Toddlers explore with their mouths; almost anything Ira could grab wound up in his mouth. An infant can be easily confined to a crib or playpen for a few moments of safety; Ira was able to climb and explore. It was time for Ira's family to take a second look at their home environment. Their pediatrician had already discussed how to store household poisons safely. For a child with multiple food allergies, having food within reach is tantamount to having poisons within reach. His parents needed to crawl around on their hands and knees, looking at their home from a different vantage point. They had placed covers over electrical outlets, but where was their food stored? They needed to childproof their house against food allergy. Easy-to-reach cabinets needed to be filled with pots and pans, which were fun to play with, while foods needed to be placed on higher shelves Ira could not reach. Meals needed to be prepared on the countertops rather than kitchen table. The garbage had to be locked in a cabinet.

In playgroups, where sharing toys and mouth-to-toy contact were common, safety precautions were also needed. Ira's family explained the issues about Ira's food allergies to the parents of the other children in these small playgroups. Toys were kept clean during the activities, and Ira's mother supervised his movements, or he was under the watchful eye of another relative or nanny who knew the issues associated with food-allergic reactions, how to prevent them, and how to treat a reaction. For trips to the mall, Ira's food was prepackaged and the family chose a clean table or used wipes to clean the chairs, Ira, and the table. The family also always had safe treats on hand for Ira. These preparations enabled him to be safe as he explored his environment.

Picky Eating

Toddlers are often finicky and have particular food preferences. They can be adamant about what they will or will not eat and sometimes do not want to eat at all. When a toddler has a food allergy and a limited diet, stubbornness can provoke anxiety in his family. Indeed, Ira could not consume milk, eggs, wheat, soy, peanuts, nuts, seafood, and seeds. His diet consisted of formula and a few fruits and vegetables, even though he was already 2 years old. He was starting to refuse particular foods, such as mashed sweet potato and fruits, and a dietitian was evaluating his diet to ensure that he was receiving appropriate nutrition. However, Ira appeared to be bored with his foods. Although the goal for a child his age is to add different foods to the diet, this is not always a successful approach, partly because young children often prefer to stay with certain food favorites of their own selection.

A number of tricks can be tried to improve the diet to make eating fun and less anxiety producing, while also providing a variety of textures and nutrients. For example, Ira was allowed to eat sweet potato but seemed to be bored with the mushy glob of potato he was served each day. I suggested some alternatives to mashed sweet potato. They could slice them into small cubes, fry them in oil safe for Ira, and let him eat these as finger foods. Longer strips of sweet potato could be used for sweet potato French fries. Sliced sweet potato pieces could be cut into fun shapes using cookie cutters and baked or fried. This strategy was applied to other foods, and mealtimes became more fun and less stressful.

Several additional approaches were used to improve mealtimes for Ira. He was allowed to choose the color of the fork to eat with. A plate with a picture at the bottom covered by his meal would surprise as him as he finished his meal. He was allowed to choose a sippy cup to be filled with his calcium-fortified rice drink or formula. Although Ira could not select what he could eat, he was able to choose the cups, plates, and utensils to use at mealtime, with pleasant surprises in store as the meal progressed successfully. When Ira became bored with one routine, his family would find new variations on a theme. They lavished him with praise and positive reinforcement for successfully trying new items and completing his meals.

When Ira was defiant, they did not fight with him about eating. Instead, they let him have some moderate control. For example, when he threw food from his plate, they would firmly state that this behavior was unacceptable, remove him from the table for a minute, and then have him return to try again. When he resumed eating, they smiled and clapped. Mealtime was not always easy; however, Ira and his family did well with this approach.

In some cases, a child's refusal to eat may be a sign of an allergic response to the food. This should be discussed with your allergist as well. For example, a child may be refusing to eat a piece of her apple because it is making her mouth itchy, which may be hard to discern. If your child spits out a particular food or refuses to try it, discuss these responses with your doctor because additional testing may be enlightening. About half the time a child refuses a food and has a positive allergy test to the food, they are found to have an allergic reaction to the food when an oral food challenge is conducted.

Childcare

Childcare for an infant or toddler with multiple food allergies requires significant preparation and flexibility by caregivers. Most childcare facilities do not have a nurse on the premises. These facilities must address the issue that if a child is eating at the site, this can pose a danger for a child with a food allergy. The challenge is particularly difficult if a child has multiple food allergies that include common foods such as milk or eggs. Depending on the age of the child and the specific activities involved, parents would need to consider exposure to shared toys. Many of the issues discussed in Chapter 22 about schools would also apply for childcare. However, some of the obstacles are much more difficult to surmount for a busy toddler who requires constant supervision. If a child is not eating in a childcare center, which is possible with part-time childcare, there may be more leeway, but if meals are taken in a childcare center, they would need to be under strict supervision with extensive cleaning up afterward. In addition, the supervising adults would need careful training about food-allergen avoidance and treatment of an allergic reaction. Resources are available through the Food Allergy & Anaphylaxis Network regarding programs for managing food allergy in childcare settings (see Part 9, "Resources").

New Allergies

For the toddler with food allergies, ages 2 to 3 or 4 is the time when new food allergies may develop, but this is also a time when certain allergies are likely to be resolved. You will certainly want to keep in contact with your pediatrician and allergist to determine whether some of the allergies have resolved, so that the diet can be adjusted accordingly. This is also a time when asthma or hay fever may develop. Upper respiratory infections, or the common cold, would be the most common reason to develop an episode of asthma. The symptoms of asthma include coughing, breathing fast, chest pulling in, or the nose flaring with breathing. Hay fever symptoms include itchy and watery eyes, nose and nasal congestion, and sneezing. If you notice these symptoms, you should discuss them promptly with your doctor. Typically, in this age group, a visit with your allergist every nine to twelve months would be recommended to evaluate food allergies and other allergic problems.

~

The first few years of life for a child with a food allergy can be challenging and rewarding. As a parent, you are called on to be creative, patient, thoughtful, and loving to make the various transitions a success, and to keep your child safe during these years. While managing your child's food allergy may be time consuming, these are years to savor because of the wonderful developments you will see in your child. Think of your child as a child, not just as a child with food allergies. Emphasizing all of the wonderful aspects of your child apart from food allergy is important for everyone and will be a major foundation on which to approach the preschool and middle-school years.

24 ~ Preschool and School-Age Children

As a child grows, he or she changes dramatically from being a pleasure-seeking, self-absorbed toddler, to a child aware of those around him. Growing up with a food allergy should not prevent your child from exploring the things that a child without food allergies would be able to explore, experience, master, and do except, of course, eating certain foods. Aiming for success during these developmental years means ensuring that your child participates in normal activities. The response to specific hurdles will vary from child to child depending on personality, the circumstances surrounding various experiences, developmental abilities, and temperament. While it may be easy to view a food allergy as an obstacle, it may also be possible to view it as an opportunity to help your child learn more about himself and others and to develop a sense of responsibility and understanding for the world around him.

Preschool

Neil is a 3½-year-old with multiple food allergies, who had already participated in a variety of playgroups and was preparing to attend preschool. Neil was becoming more aware of those around him and aware that he was different because he could not eat some of the foods other children enjoyed. His family wanted more information about how they could help him to get ready for school. They had already discussed Neil's needs with the school. Other students at the school had food allergies as well, including Neil's cousin, Garrett. Therefore, the school had plans in place that could reasonably help ensure Neil's safety.

Independence

Neil was at that age in which he was able to explore his environment at will. This meant that Neil could potentially take another child's food or find a way to obtain unsafe food at home. Neil was able to tolerate soy but was not allowed to have any milk products. He had his emergency action plan and medications nearby at all times. Neil's parents had always told Neil about his food allergies and he seemed to understand, but now he had questions about these allergies too. How should the family present his allergies to Neil?

I suggested that they use certain words to describe food allergy to Neil. It is not a good idea to discuss potentially fatal reactions with a young child. Death is a difficult concept for preschoolers to grasp. I recommend that families tell their child that certain foods can make them "sick" if they eat them and that mom and dad would not want him to be sick. Use simple but direct words when discussing those foods that can be eaten or must be avoided. For example, families may get into the habit of calling an allergic child's drink "milk," even though it may not actually be cow's milk. This may cause confusion when a child is around other children. For example, the other children are drinking "milk" and Neil would be drinking "milk," but Neil's milk was actually a soy drink or a rice drink. Begin early to call the food by its proper name. For example, Neil's "soy drink" or Neil's "safe soy milk."

Because Neil's parents would be monitoring his actions less, it was also important for him to learn about his safe foods and the individuals who would be responsible for providing safe food. A young child should not be solely responsible for selecting foods or judging who may be able to provide safe foods; it may be easier to teach your child that certain individuals will know which foods would be safe for him to eat. For example, if Neil spent time with an aunt knowledgeable about his allergies, he would know that his aunt would be responsible for selecting his safe foods. Neil would be reminded that specific people provide safe foods for him, such as his parents and aunt. However, he would also be reminded that other individuals may offer him food, but he should refuse. While there are many variations on how to introduce these concepts to your child, a simple explanation is best: "There are many delicious foods that are safe for you, Neil, and mom or dad will provide these safe foods. It would not be safe and could make you sick if you took food from any other children or adults, other than from your aunt or us. Your lunch and snack are in your lunchbox that has your name and this sticker with your picture on it." Neil was also told about special nonperishable snacks and foods kept for him by his teacher in a special box at school. These would be available and safe for him to eat and could be used in case he forgot lunch or if there was a classroom celebration involving food.

I have also suggested that families test their child to assess a child's capabilities. It is not always obvious what a child's view on life may be until parents ask. For example, you may tell a child not to go with strangers and find out that your child's definition of a stranger does not match your own. Similarly, teaching your child not to take food from others may be overridden by a child's trust in an adult. If your child will be in a situation in which he may be offered foods from others, set up a situation you supervise as a test. For example, have a friend or relative offer your child a cookie while you watch. How will your child react? Will she ask you if it is okay? Will she take the cookie because she knows and trusts the adult? By practicing these scenarios, teaching the right responses, giving positive reinforcement and only gently disapproving for wrong decisions, and repeating these training sessions occasionally, you will reinforce competence and confidence in your child. Of course, you will want to ensure safety through other means not under your child's control. Although you will want to teach your child not to take food from others, you will certainly still teach those around your child not to offer unsafe foods.

Preschool

The good news about this age group is the tremendous and rapid progress made between ages 3 and 5 in children's understanding of allergies and their ability to protect themselves. But depending on the specific developmental abilities of your child, preschool, kindergarten, and first-grade years can be particularly challenging if your child does not recognize specific boundaries or is likely to continue to explore items orally. With other children around, sharing toys that wind up in children's mouths means toys will need to be frequently cleaned and separated. Your child's caregiver would need to ensure that items are free from food residues, which may require, for example, wiping the toys that are going to be placed into the mouth. Many of the issues described in Chapter 22 about managing a food allergy in school would, of course, apply to a preschool child. Because the child is less in control of herself and her environment, additional safety measures must be considered.

Of course, only safe meals would be planned for school, typically safe foods prepared by you for your child. The preschool-age child is receptive to learning about her food allergy. This educational opportunity can be extended to your child's classmates. Videos available through the Food Allergy & Anaphylaxis Network and books for children will teach that a food may be fine for some children but make other children ill. The symptoms of an allergic reaction can be described in nonthreatening ways to children in this age group, so that they will learn to recognize reactions in themselves or others. This type of teaching also provides your child's classmates with the age-appropriate knowledge to empathize with your child.

Showing your child the medications you carry on her behalf is also important. Your child should know about these medications, but, of course, you would not want them to hold the self-injectable epinephrine without your supervision. It should always be clear that trained adults who supervise your child are responsible for keeping your child safe. But your child also has a role to play in not sharing foods with others, only eating the foods that are known to be safe, and telling adults of any symptoms or problems. Not every child in this age group will understand the specifics of safe or unsafe food, the symptoms of an allergic reaction, or the use of medications. However, this limitation should not prevent you from introducing these concepts, which will be developed over time. This might be the time for your child to wear medical identification jewelry since she will be spending more time away from you.

New and Resolving Food Allergies and Other Allergies

The highest rate for outgrowing milk, eggs, wheat, or soy allergies occurs during preschool. Children may also outgrow allergies to peanuts, nuts, or seafood. Discuss further testing and possibly expanding the diet with your pediatrician and allergist. This is also the time when allergic rhinitis symptoms—itchy, watery eyes and a runny, itchy nose—are likely to develop because your child has lived through a few pollen seasons. Because the risk for these allergies increases, you should be aware of these symptoms. Altering the environment or using medications can treat them. For the preschool-age child who must concentrate on schoolwork, treating these allergic symptoms means fewer distractions for your child and a chance to enjoy school.

The School-Age Child

You and your child face new challenges with each passing year, as your child moves from kindergarten through eighth grade and prepares for high school. A child learns more about the world around him and may begin to recognize the effect of having food allergy. He may express feelings about the limitations that living with a food allergy imposes. However, these life experiences are also an opportunity for more discussion and learning. The school-aged child can take on more responsibility, learn about his food allergies, understand others, and continue to participate in school activities.

School

Wendy is a fourth-grader who has milk, peanut, and tree nut allergies. She had been eating at a peanut-free table with several selected friends since first grade. However, she was pressuring her family to let her eat at the regular table with the other children. Her parents wanted more advice about this.

Indeed, many issues about food allergy will arise as a child gets older. When Wendy was in the first and second grades, she was somewhat impulsive and would often grab food from others. Therefore, a designated "allergy table," with increased supervision and exclusion of some of the foods she was allergic to was a good solution. However, as a fourth-grader, she controlled and understood her own food allergies, and it was clear to her, and to her parents and school personnel, that she could safely eat the foods that she brought from home. Casual contact exposure for Wendy was not considered a significant issue. Even if milk had spilled on her, she knew to wash off the spill. The expectation was that such an exposure would unlikely result in a severe reaction. Considering the social issues and Wendy's ability to protect herself, it was agreed that joining her classmates during lunchtime made sense.

Self-management of an allergy changes through the school-age years. Depending on your child's own abilities, changes in a care plan can occur that match what your child is capable of doing to keep safe. For example, some young children may not be depended on to hold their own emergency medications because they may injure themselves or others by playing with them or the child may not understand when or how to use them. As a child progresses through grade school, she may be more likely to understand these medications, be able to safely carry them with her, and potentially administer them, if needed. Of course, even if your child is well-trained, there should always be a responsible adult nearby to evaluate and treat an allergic reaction.

Other children can be cruel during these years, and it is important to watch out for and to confront bullying immediately. Help your child understand the importance of telling an adult about bullying and that he is not a tattle-tale for doing so. Educating classmates about food allergies, their seriousness, and the dangerous repercussions of bullying may reduce that behavior. Books and videos available through the Food Allergy & Anaphylaxis Network (Part 9) can aid in this educational process.

Because of peer pressure at school, your child may be tempted to eat unsafe food. Talk to your child about peer pressure. Ask questions: How would you respond if someone asked you to eat something unsafe? Help your child formulate his answers before the situation arises. This is the age at which body self-awareness occurs, and your child will be able to tell you or others about allergy symptoms. Gently explain the symptoms individuals may experience during an allergic reaction and that your child must inform others promptly about symptoms. Sometimes a child may be afraid to notify an adult if he "cheated" on his diet. It may be useful to tell him that you trust and count on him to eat safely, but if he ever made a bad choice and developed symptoms, he must still tell an adult. He would be in more trouble if he waited or did not let an adult know. Encourage your child to be honest and forthcoming about symptoms or dietary indiscretions.

Home

Time at home with your school-aged child is a perfect opportunity to teach independence about food allergy and safety. She should understand, in an age-appropriate way, exactly how and when to use her emergency medications. Allow your child to practice with a trainer device. She should be encouraged to carry the medication, to wear medical identification jewelry, and to know about obtaining safe foods. Compliment her accomplishments. Sometimes children do not want to wear the medical identification bracelets. Find a way to make wearing it interesting or fun; change the type of jewelry occasionally, or use fashionable or sporty bracelets.

This is also the age group in which shopping for safe foods should be an opportunity for teaching your child what is involved in reading labels and obtaining safe foods. You might start with games such as, "Wendy, read this label . . . Is this food safe for you?" This is also the age in which independence in obtaining a restaurant meal could be taught. For example, have your child practice telling a waiter about her allergies and help her order a safe meal in a restaurant. This exercise not only stresses independence but also identifies tools needed to eat safely. Prepare a list of questions, with your child's help, for your allergist or pediatrician. In this way, she will be taking an active part in her own healthcare. Children may have questions you did not think of. Let your child formulate and ask the questions.

While the preschool and school ages pose new challenges in keeping your child safe, numerous opportunities exist to help your child understand his allergy and to control his environment. These tools can be learned easily at this point and will be incredibly important as your child becomes an independent high school student.

25 ~ Teenagers and Young Adults

When 14-year-old Helene entered high school, she was more concerned with making new friends and fitting in than with her food allergies. Helene had peanut and tree nut allergies and had experienced a severe allergic reaction when she was 5 years old. Since then, her family had been careful to ensure that she had no further exposures to peanuts or tree nuts and maintained a strict emergency care plan. Helene never needed any medications for allergic reactions over the years. She had little recollection of allergic reactions other than she was not allowed to have particular foods. Her family brought her to see me because they were concerned she was not taking her allergies seriously and might eat recklessly and perhaps not have her medications available.

Indeed Helene's parents have valid concerns. The teenage years can be a particularly risky time for those with life-threatening food allergies. In studies about fatalities from food-induced anaphylaxis, teenagers and young adults with food allergies make up a disproportionate number of deaths. In one series of thirty-two fatalities, 69 percent of the fatalities were children aged 11 to 21 years. Almost all of these individuals had a known diagnosis of food allergy and asthma and had experienced previous reactions. However, fewer than 10 percent had epinephrine at the time of the reaction. Our research group, in collaboration with the Food Allergy & Anaphylaxis Network, has undertaken a variety of studies to learn more about why adolescence is a risky time for severe food-allergic reactions.

In one study, we asked parents and their teenaged children similar questions. All of the teenagers had been prescribed epinephrine. Only half of the parents thought that their teenager would be responsible for self-administering medications, but 73 percent of the teenagers indicated that they would (100 percent would have been ideal). This finding was important because we also learned that to ensure that teenagers feel comfortable and empowered to self-administer medication they need to understand how and when to do so.

When parents were asked their fears about their child's food allergy, the parents of teens typically feared their child would have a severe reaction or die. However, teenagers were worried about the social isolation, and 94 percent indicated that this was the hardest part about having a food allergy. Teenagers see themselves as immortal. This feeling of immortality, combined with social pressure and a need to fit in, may explain why the teenage years can be risky for food allergies. Risk taking may increase because the teenager does not fear the consequences or believes he can control the consequences.

With funding from the Food Allergy Initiative and work of the Food Allergy & Anaphylaxis Network, we undertook an additional survey of 174 teenagers and young adults with a variety of food allergies. Three out of 4 teenagers indicated that they always carry their epinephrine; however, in reality the frequency of carrying varied, depending on their activities. When teenagers travel or eat out, many carried their epinephrine with them, probably because their parents were with them. However, only two-thirds had the medication with them when they were at friends' homes or at school activities. The number of teens who carried their epinephrine with them decreased, depending on certain social activities. For example, only 43 percent carried epinephrine with them when they were participating in sporting activities, and if they were wearing tight clothing, only half had their epinephrine with them. It is apparent that social circumstances affect whether a teenager carries his medication.

The study results remind parents to ensure that their teenagers understand the importance of having the medication available, including at sporting events, even if it is unlikely they will be eating. We identified a higher-risk group among teenagers. These teens were less likely to have medications with them or to read ingredient labels. Indeed, we found that this high-risk group was less concerned with their allergy and more likely to indicate that they felt "different" than others because of their allergy. These findings may be expected because these teenagers reflect a lower-perceived risk of allergy and perhaps a stronger desire to blend in with children on unrestricted diets. Although not all of the teens reported that they explained their allergies to their friends, most felt that educating their friends would make living with food allergies easier.

How can we use the results of these studies to help protect Helene and other teenagers with life-threatening food allergies? Helene and I spoke privately about her allergies and whether she followed the rules, read labels, made healthy food choices, and carried emergency medications. Helene admitted that she often did not take her medications with her when she thought that she would not be eating anything. She was a bit embarrassed to discuss food allergy with her friends, but some of her best friends knew about her food allergy. She was always careful to only eat foods when she had read the ingredient label carefully. On the few occasions she had opportunities to eat with others in a restaurant, she did not feel comfortable explaining her allergies to the restaurant staff. Instead she ordered foods she assumed would be safe.

I explained that sometimes a food-allergic reaction could happen even though she expected not to eat. For example, a spontaneous trip to a restaurant might lead Helene to eat a food that appears safe but is not. A better approach, I explained, would be to carry her medications at all times, something she could accomplish easily because she usually carried a purse or backpack. (For boys, I would often explain that a belt clip, large pocket in cargo pants, or backpack would be a good choice to conveniently carry medications.) Helene and I reviewed the use of self-administered epinephrine, and she practiced with this medicine using a trainer device. We also agreed that we would try to inform her friends how to help her if she were in need. Helene had been wearing a medical identification bracelet, for which she was commended.

I then met with Helene and her parents to discuss the various studies of teen behavior. It was natural for Helene to feel peer pressure and to not always want to have her medications with her. However, we agreed that Helene's parents would continue to remind her about carrying her medications with her and would review the steps necessary to acquire safe foods. I do not like to scare children or their parents during office visits, but I did explain that Helene was at risk for a severe allergic reaction, a potentially fatal one, because of her age, her specific allergies, and her asthma. We discussed how it was important to keep her asthma under control, and I also explained that teenagers' fatal reactions usually occurred when they had delayed getting treatment for their symptoms. Some teenagers would go off to their room or into an isolated location hoping their symptoms would pass, when, in fact, symptoms worsened and they were unable to get help. I stressed that Helene's parents would remind her about carrying her medications because they love her, not because they were trying to annoy or harass her.

In addition to keep Helene safe, it was going to be important to educate her friends and others about her allergies. The Food Allergy & Anaphylaxis

Network has a program called Protect A Life, or PAL, that educates family and friends on how to assist loved ones with allergies. Often, positive peer pressure reinforces healthy practices for a young person with food allergies. The Food Allergy & Anaphylaxis Network also has a Web site and newsletter for teenagers that I recommended to Helene.

Because Helene was shy about talking to restaurant waitstaff about her food allergies, I suggested she practice with her family. One parent would introduce the issue to the restaurant server and Helene would join in and question the server about the menu. She would also shop for groceries with her family to prepare for college. We talked about dating, in particular, kissing a partner who had eaten a food allergen and how to avoid the risk. Helene and her parents also informed friends, teachers, and coaches about her food allergies.

Helene seemed receptive, and her parents were excited about giving her more responsibility and independence. But, a concern remained. Helene played soccer, and because her teammates generally did not bring food to practice, she thought it was unnecessary to carry epinephrine or explain her food allergies to her coach and teammates. So I asked her to consider the following scenario: She's on the field. A teammate who had just eaten a peanut butter sandwich sips out of her water bottle unbeknown to her. After practice, she drinks from the water bottle and has an allergic reaction. She has no epinephrine and, to make matters worse, her teammates and coach have no idea what's happening to her. Although this scenario seemed far-fetched, Helene and her parents accepted that the plans had to be applied in all circumstances.

Over the ensuing years, reports about Helene's progress were encouraging. Her class held a program about food allergies, and Helene taught the class about safe meal preparation for people with food allergies. Several of her closest friends became some of her strongest advocates, always ensuring that Helene had her medications when they traveled together and ensuring that restaurant staff paid extra special attention to make certain that she was obtaining safe foods. Her parents began to see Helene's food allergy less as a handicap. It made Helene stronger, and by Helene's senior year, she felt that way too. She was well on her way to being able to maintain a safe lifestyle at college.

The teenage years can be filled with defiant behaviors. Not every teenager has an easy path like Helene. However, parents must ensure that a teenager's friends and teachers understand food allergy. Frustrations and difficulties will occur along the way, but patience and understanding should prevail. Talk to your child about allergies the way you would talk about drugs or alcohol. The point is to keep an open line of communication and always listen carefully when your teenager indicates something is bothering him.

Young Adults

I met 18-year-old David and his family a month before he went to college. David had experienced several food-allergic reactions to tree nuts and shellfish during high school. He had experienced several reactions at restaurants with his friends, and it was apparent he did not make a strong effort to obtain safe meals. He often did not carry his emergency medications with him, although he had been prescribed self-injectable epinephrine. Several of the reactions that he had experienced were fairly mild, but some included vomiting and wheezing, and once he apparently lost consciousness. He generally treated his symptoms with antihistamines. He had not told his family about two of the more serious reactions but confided to me when we spoke privately. His family was concerned about college because they already felt that he was taking too many risks by not taking his allergies seriously.

David believed because he had never had a severe reaction or an emergency room visit, his allergy was not worrisome. David had generally not prepared his own meals. His family provided him with safe foods. Thus, most reactions had occurred from foods he had obtained on his own, from other children, or when eating out. He had medical identification jewelry, but generally did not wear it, and only a few of his friends knew about his food allergies. The family had not contacted the college ahead of time about David's food allergies; they came to my office to satisfy the college's request for information about David's allergies.

We had to ensure that David was prepared for a safe college experience. The issues that were successfully addressed with Helene when she was 14 were unaddressed for David during high school. We talked about the seriousness of his allergy, the pitfalls that he had already experienced, and how lucky he was to have survived some of the allergic reactions. I explained how reactions can vary from time to time and may be mild at some times and severe at others. Even individuals who had not experienced a severe allergic reaction could be at risk for a deadly reaction. That he was eating dangerously, did not carry the appropriate medications, or did not use them when he needed to, were potentially life-threatening circumstances.

We reviewed how and when to use self-injectable epinephrine. We also reviewed how meals could be obtained safely and talked about the importance of alerting friends and individuals at the school about his allergies. Because he would be eating his meals in the college cafeteria, we needed to inform the school about safe meal provisions in the cafeteria. A lot of time had been lost for David. We needed to move quickly to help him acquire safe foods on his own, including at restaurants, and to ensure that an emergency action plan was in place at his school. I was particularly concerned about alcohol or drug use and how these could impair his judgment. This was also discussed openly.

I arranged for David to see an allergist close to his college. As it turned out, David's school had a variety of plans in place for individuals with food allergies so obtaining a safe meal would not be difficult. The school health service was open to helping David manage his allergies. With his permission, the school health service paired David with two other college students who had food allergies. With careful follow-up and frequent discussions with the school health center, the allergist, and his family, David's safety was maximized even with the late start.

The teenage years and young adulthood represent a special time of risk for children because they must take responsibility for their own safety and, at the same time, face peer pressure and their feelings of immortality. By constantly engaging these young individuals, keeping an open line of communication, and involving those around them, it is possible to improve day-to-day safety, promote good habits, and help them to successfully manage life with a food allergy.

PART 6

EMOTIONAL CONCERNS

Living with food allergy is a significant challenge. We have performed several studies on the effect of food allergy on quality of life. The illness affects every aspect of life for the allergic child and family. Whether it is shopping; being with relatives and friends, at school or camp; or maintaining diligence at every meal, food allergies affect life. The effect on quality of life, according to the studies we have performed in collaboration with the Food Allergy & Anaphylaxis Network for families with a food-allergic child, is similar to the experience of families with children with chronic diseases such as rheumatoid arthritis or diabetes.

In Part 6, several of the common emotional problems that arise for families with a child with food allergies are discussed and some solutions are offered. In many situations, simply recognizing the effect that food allergy may have on the individual and the family is an important step in overcoming problems. Understanding the root of these issues is a major goal of Part 6. While this topic emphasizes many of the difficulties encountered in living with food allergies, the positive side must not be forgotten. Families and individuals living with food allergies also describe feelings of increased responsibility, emotional fortitude, and personal growth. These positive outcomes must also be acknowledged.

26 ~ The Effect on Children and Families

Fourteen-year-old Melanie had food allergies to peanuts, tree nuts, seeds, fish, and shellfish. She also had milk, egg, and soy allergies, which she had outgrown. She had experienced approximately a dozen reactions over her lifetime, including three anaphylactic reactions. Her last reaction occurred at age 11, when she ate a sesame seed bagel. Melanie had become fearful of eating, particularly for the previous six months before her parents brought her to my office. Over the past year, she had cut down significantly on the variety and quantity of foods she was willing to eat, fearful of an allergic reaction. In private conversation with Melanie, she indicated that she was satisfied with her current diet, albeit it was very restricted, and she felt safer keeping her diet isolated to a narrow choice of safe foods. When I spoke with her parents, it was evident that Melanie expressed anxiety about having another allergic reaction but was unwilling to eat foods she tolerated. She had lost a lot of weight in the preceding six months, having limited her diet to about ten foods, and she showed disinterest in eating.

For Melanie's family, food had always been a major point of discussion and anxiety. They felt that they had been fairly successful over Melanie's lifetime in preventing reactions and responding to reactions when they occurred, but everyone in the family acknowledged that the process had become more difficult for the past several years. Melanie's 7-year-old brother, Steven, had become aware of how his life was affected by Melanie's allergies. Steven complained that "everything was always about Melanie," and he admitted that sometimes he would like to give foods to Melanie to make her sick. Melanie's mother complained that the she carried the burden of keeping Melanie safe, that Melanie's father did not understand the significance of Melanie's allergy, and that several of the allergic reactions had occurred while he and Melanie were together. The family was experiencing more than their share of the emotional stress associated with food allergies.

Fear and Anxiety

Living with a life-threatening food allergy poses a source of fear and anxiety, at least three times a day with each meal and possibly many more times when snacks and social situations are considered. Three adverse emotional or psychological responses may emerge for individuals with significant allergies. One pattern of behavior is *food refusal.* When eating focuses on safety, the experience of eating may become less pleasurable and provokes anxiety. Even toddlers may refuse new foods or foods they had previously eaten, thereby narrowing their repertoire of choices.

Another related problem is *generalization of reactions.* For example, a child may have experienced allergic reactions to several foods and then begins to complain of problems, usually of a mild nature, from a variety of other foods. This can be a tricky circumstance because it is always possible that the child is truly experiencing actual allergic reactions and is developing allergies to other foods but often this is not the case. In some instances, it may be clear that mild allergic symptoms from another cause are being attributed to food. For example, a child may have hay fever, with sneezing and mouth itchiness. The child may attribute these symptoms to various meals, which limits the diet. A *panic response,* the third potential outcome, can be misunderstood as an allergic reaction. Some children have had severe reactions to foods, and this can result in a posttraumatic stress disorder, like individuals who have gone to war and come back traumatized, where if they hear a loud noise they may want to hide under the table, thinking that they are still in battle. For such children, panic responses can mimic allergic reactions.

Melanie had fear and anxiety because of food. On one occasion, Melanie had a panic attack that mimicked a food-allergic reaction. About a year before her visit with me, Melanie was sitting with friends who were sharing a bag of potato chips. Melanie thought that the potato chips smelled funny and asked her friends to check the ingredient label; the potato chips contained peanut oil. Melanie experienced heart racing, sweating, difficulty breathing, and finger numbness. She was treated for an allergic reaction; however, it was unlikely she had experienced a true allergic reaction. First, she had not actually eaten the potato chips, so a severe allergic reaction was unlikely. Second, it was later disclosed that the peanut oil in the potato chips was a highly processed peanut oil, which would not have contained any peanut protein. Therefore, Melanie had not been exposed to peanuts. Her symptoms, although they shared features with a true allergic reaction, were classic anxiety, or panic attack.

I explained to Melanie's family that these symptoms are not completely unexpected in someone who has experienced a significant allergic reaction. Many people are familiar with the experiment of Pavlov's dogs, where ringing a bell and feeding the dogs were performed simultaneously on a number of occasions, and then when the bell rang when food was not present, the dog would salivate. Although salivation is not a conscious response, these dogs had learned that the sound of the bell meant that they would be fed. Melanie's assumption about the potato chip having peanut resulted in significant symptoms, albeit these were anxiety symptoms. This response could be considered a natural protective response, simply a fear from something that you know, or think, can hurt you.

My first step to help Melanie was to discuss with her and her family the possibility that she refused foods because of her fears of allergic reactions. For individuals who overgeneralize reactions to foods, I usually recommend oral food challenges. By using a double-blinded, placebo-controlled food challenge method, a panic response is reduced because the child and the observers do not know when the food allergen is being tested. Through these tests, I have been able to help children expand their diet and overcome fear responses to food. Sometimes people with food allergies who happen to have symptoms from hay fever or asthma worry that their symptoms are actually caused by foods. Discussing the circumstances of these symptoms with an allergist is often all that is needed to allay concerns.

For young children with food refusal, it is often necessary for parents to be very persistent to reward small gains and to also know when not to push too hard. Some families develop reward systems when their children try new foods or finish meals. For example, place a sticker on a chart each time your child eats a new food and after a certain number of stickers are collected give your child a book or a small toy. These types of behavioral programs can be helpful in overcoming simple problematic behaviors associated with eating but must be age appropriate. Obviously, a sticker chart would not be appropriate for Melanie, but for younger children, these simple reward systems can be very effective.

When starting out with a reward system like this, rewards should be given for any level of success. For example, an award would be given for taking an extra bite of a food or trying a bite of one new food, and as time goes by, the rewards could be given for larger gains. The system must be simple for younger children but can be more complex as children grow up. For example, a trip to a movie may be the reward for two weeks of appropriate behaviors for an older child. Of course, if you have reason to believe your child is allergic to a food you would like him to eat, do not force him. Discuss your concerns with your allergist first. Sometimes when anxiety is strong, reward systems are not enough. For Melanie, who had significantly altered the world around her, more work had to be done.

Depression and Sadness

Melanie was not generally unhappy, but she expressed sadness about her food allergies and wished that she did not have them. Her mother had become depressed with her family situation. Melanie continued to exclude more and more foods from her diet. It is common to see these types of feelings in individuals with food allergies and their family members. When these experiences are mild and transient, and do not impede day-to-day activities, I generally explain to families that these are natural feelings that should be acknowledged. Many families seek and obtain comfort by discussing what they are going through with other families in similar circumstances. Large organizations like the Food Allergy & Anaphylaxis Network and also many local organizations such as parents groups, support groups, or smaller associations provide opportunities for families to get together and discuss living with food allergy. By sharing their experiences, many people understand that some level of depression or sadness is normal but that they can also overcome depression and sadness to enjoy their lives and family.

However, some families become crippled from the frustrations of living with food allergy and become depressed to a degree that they do not enjoy life. Apart from the food allergy, individuals may suffer from depression. Seeking professional help from psychologists, psychiatrists, or counselors is important. Although it is not likely that food allergy would result in depression that would need medication, it is certainly possible to have depression that is exacerbated by food allergy, and both counseling and medication might be needed. In my evaluation of Melanie and her family, clinical depression was not apparent, but sadness and frustration were, brought on by Melanie's refusal to eat a varied diet and weight loss. We discussed these issues openly, which helped as the family began to acknowledge their feelings more.

Guilt

Melanie's mother blamed herself for causing Melanie's allergies because she ate peanuts and fish during pregnancy and breast-feeding. Melanie's father blamed himself for allergic reactions that occurred in his presence. Melanie felt guilty for "causing all of the problems in her family." Guilt is sometimes a natural consequence in families with food allergies. As human beings, we want to find reasons for our experiences, and when it is difficult to find a reason, it is easy to blame oneself or others. It is very common for parents to feel that they have caused their child's food allergy through their own diet. As Chapter 29 indicates, there is no clear evidence that ingesting certain foods during breast-feeding or pregnancy contributes to childhood allergies.

In many situations, recognizing that the allergies are "nobody's fault" helps to open up lines of communication to reduce guilt, and this was immediately apparent when I discussed these issues with Melanie's mother and the rest of the members of the family. It was neither Melanie's fault that she had food allergies nor her mother's fault. Her father had made a few mistakes but understood now what was involved in keeping Melanie safe and could move on. If guilt feelings are overwhelming and are affecting family activities, discussing the problem with your doctor or seeking professional help are advised.

Sibling Rivalry

Melanie and Steven were seven years apart, and although Steven felt jealous of the attention Melanie received and Melanie felt guilty for causing stress in the family, they were only experiencing a modest amount of sibling rivalry. The main rivalry was attention from their parents. Because of Melanie's allergies, much of the attention was aimed toward Melanie and her food allergies. This was particularly the situation in the preceding six months because she had lost weight and was limiting her diet more significantly. In many situations, children who are closer in age will experience more issues of sibling rivalry. This is not unique to food allergy and can occur in any illness that may take up a lot of the family's time and attention, and it is essentially a natural outcome of the need to give additional attention to the ill child. However, with food allergies, an additional problem arises because dietary restrictions may be applied to all family meals, which affect the nonallergic family members.

In some families where several children may have food allergies, rivalries result because the child with more foods eliminated may receive more attention. In all of these situations, the primary helpful response is to acknowledge the problem. I have seen families very successfully address sibling rivalry through open communication and that these feelings are natural and are not rooted in hate. By establishing that all of the children in the family are loved, and by making special accommodations that acknowledge the child without food allergies, anxieties can be overcome. For example, earlier in Melanie and Steven's childhood, the family had taken special picnics to Steven's favorite park. Melanie was included in all of the activities and had special foods to eat, but Steven was the focus. He selected the activities for the day and was given special attention during that time.

Anger and Frustration

Living with food allergy causes some degree of anger and frustration. Although Melanie and her family were currently experiencing feelings of sadness and guilt, they also acknowledged that through the years there had been many periods of rather extreme anger. Melanie was often angry about her allergies. Her mother was angry and frustrated that she could not "make it all go away" and often became frustrated with the constant and unending tasks to keep Melanie healthy. The family sometimes felt punished. Everyone remembered times they cried or had emotional outbursts.

Many families find comfort in simply knowing that they are not alone. Sometimes families do not communicate feelings, and they fester. Open communication within the family is important so that these emotions can be acknowledged. When Melanie was 7 years old, her mother found her punching a pillow because she was angry that she could not eat peanut butter like her best friend. Her mother reminded her that her friend was mad that Melanie could whistle, but her friend could not. This acknowledgment made Melanie feel better. Sometimes anger is associated with a particular situation; in this case, finding a solution to the problem may reduce the anger. When Melanie was feeling angry about a school field trip that included a visit to a candy factory with free samples, her mother was able to arrange for an alternative snack treat from the same factory. Of course, not every problem can be solved. Many families or individuals with food allergies find comfort in sharing their experiences with others who also have food allergies. It is helpful to know that feelings of anger and frustration are common and can be overcome. Many families have found that simply discussing the anger, moving on to solve problems when possible, and accentuating positive experiences and successes provide all that is needed to lessen anger and frustration. However, if anger and frustration affect daily life, professional help from a psychologist or counselor might be in order.

Spouses and Relatives

Melanie's parents had become distant over the preceding years and blamed much of their marital strife on managing Melanie and her food allergies. Her parents felt blame, guilt, anger, and frustration. Melanie's mother was upset with her husband who seemed not to take the allergies seriously and seemed to separate himself from the anger and arguments between Melanie and her mother about her diet. Melanie's father felt his wife was consumed with Melanie's allergies and her food issues and did not pay enough attention to him and to other aspects of the home.

Anxieties and frustrations over chronic illness in a family can take their toll on spousal relationships and relationships with other relatives. I encourage families to approach food allergy early on as an issue for the entire family. When one spouse does not seem to take the allergy seriously, both parents should meet with the doctor, apart from the child, to pose questions and clear up misconceptions. It was evident that Melanie's parents were dealing with other marital problems, so I recommended additional counseling for them as a couple.

Putting It All Together

As I learned more about Melanie and her family, I became concerned that Melanie had anorexia nervosa and that she was limiting her diet because of this illness, using her food allergy to explain her actions to her family and herself. Melanie had misperceptions about her body proportions and expressed stronger concerns about these issues than about her food allergies. I referred her family for psychiatric evaluation, and, indeed, Melanie was diagnosed with anorexia nervosa and underwent treatment for this disorder. Regarding the food allergy, her parents and I came up with an appropriate level of avoidance for peanuts, tree nuts, seeds, fish, and shellfish. The family received marital and family counseling to help as Melanie faced this significant mental health diagnosis. Her family did well with the additional counseling.

Living with food allergy can affect quality of life in different ways. Many unhappy emotions are normal, expected responses to stress and illness. Living with a food allergy can be like living in a field of land mines, where any meal can cause a problem. Living and managing this situation can lead to fear, anxiety, sadness, depression, anger, frustration, guilt, rivalry among siblings, and stress between spouses and other family members. If these problems arise, or even before they do, the issues must be addressed. Children who have experienced an allergic reaction can be fearful about exposure to foods and eating, a problem that needs to be acknowledged and treated, usually by consulting with an allergist, pediatrician, and other families. However, when emotional problems disrupt a child's enjoyment of life or when harmony suffers, professional help from psychologists, counselors, and psychiatrists is crucial.

27 ~ Maintaining a Healthy Lifestyle

Allan is a 6-year-old with peanut and tree nut allergies whose parents had imposed strict avoidance measures in his day-to-day life. Allan had experienced a mild allergic reaction to peanut at age 1 when he was diagnosed with peanut allergy. At age 3, he had his first accidental exposure to peanut, which resulted in a significant reaction requiring an emergency room visit. Thereafter, various restrictions were applied to Allan's lifestyle. The family had already excluded peanut and tree nut items from their home. Their two other children were not allowed to eat any peanut or tree nut products at home or outside of the home, even though Allan's older siblings previously had been eating peanut and tree nut products. Initially, Allan was participating in playgroups, but his family became fearful that he might touch or eat something with peanut, so he no longer participated in playgroups. Allan's family invited children from the neighborhood to their home from the time Allan was 3 or 4 years old, but they would ask the other families to ensure that their children had not eaten peanut for a day before coming to their home, and many of the families were reluctant about sending their children to Allan's home. Allan's family imposed more limitations on what Allan was allowed to do to avoid any peanut exposures. Although he had been going to playgrounds and shopping centers and malls, these activities were curtailed, and Allan was spending more time at home.

Allan's parents considered home schooling him. The family curtailed summer travel and limited their recreation activities to brief trips because they did not feel comfortable choosing food for Allan in restaurants. Besides, they undertook extreme cleaning procedures at hotels, so vacations were not enjoyable. Family members agreed that protecting Allan was a priority; however, stress was rising because Allan's allergies imposed limitations on everyone's lifestyle.

Avoiding Seclusion

Individuals with food allergies should be able to participate in all of the usual activities of life, except that they cannot ingest the food to which they are allergic. While exposure through casual contact is an issue for some, particularly younger children, most individuals with food allergy should be able to participate in daily activities safely. Home schooling is an excellent choice for many families; however, home schooling should not be pursued solely to avoid exposure to avoided foods.

Allan's family had taken increasing measures to exclude any possibility of Allan coming into contact with the food to which he was allergic. When they came to me for evaluation, they had questions about the severity of his allergy and whether they were doing enough to keep him away from peanuts. Many strategies can be implemented to ensure a safe environment, and strategies are aimed at maintaining a safe and healthy lifestyle. One outcome of food allergy is seclusion from day-to-day life. This is certainly an outcome to be avoided. The first step in addressing these issues is to discuss the realities of the risks of exposures with a trusted allergist or pediatrician.

I reviewed with Allan's family the issue of casual contact and whether what they were doing was age appropriate or necessary for Allan, considering that he had an excellent understanding of his peanut allergy and seemed to be at very low risk of having any significant reactions from casual exposures. His parents had overgeneralized their exclusion tactics. I performed some simple tests with Allan. He touched peanuts, which showed that he was fine with this level of exposure. We talked about ways to reintroduce Allan to interactions with friends and relatives and eventually to participating in school and camp. It was not a good approach to throw him into every social situation from which he had been excluded, so a step-by-step approach was agreed on. By understanding the issue and looking at the solution in small steps, there was much less anxiety associated with Allan's peanut allergy. It was important for Allan's independence that he participate in activities with other children and gradually take some responsibility for his allergies, which would benefit him in the long run.

General Well-Being

Food allergies occur among individuals and families with every type of personality and every type of family structure. Families and individuals handle problems, whether food allergy or any other issues such as death of a relative, terminal illness, financial stress, or other life stresses, in a host of different ways. Some families or individuals seem to attack adversity head-on and emerge happy and victorious, while others may be downtrodden by similar challenges. With food allergy or other stresses of life, emerging with a general feeling of health and well-being is important. The way to achieve those goals will vary depending on many circumstances. In our studies on quality of life of families living with a child who has food allergies there was a significant adverse effect on perceived general health and well-being. For children who do not have chronic daily disease but have a life-threatening food allergy, there is often discord between what outsiders see and what a family living with this illness experiences. The family's daily quality of life is negatively affected by constant vigilance to avoid the food allergen.

Despite the challenges, one step toward maintaining a state of well-being is to recognize and emphasize the positive. Families managing food allergies must remain aware of health risks, but they must also understand that, in every other way, children with food allergies are generally healthy and should be able to lead happy and productive lives. If the effect of living with a food allergy becomes overwhelming or affects day-to-day activities, like it had for Allan's family, address concerns with your physicians, including your allergist and pediatrician whose advice may be geared to your own circumstances. They may suggest that you seek help by sharing your experiences with other families. In some circumstances, counselors, psychologists, or psychiatrists should be consulted to ensure a general state of happiness and well-being.

Seeking Help for Specific Problems

Allan was doing well after the family had gradually reintroduced him to a more open lifestyle of play dates, visits to the park and shopping malls, and eventually school and camp. By the time Allan was 9 years old, he was enjoying many social activities with his friends. However, his family had developed certain concerns about Allan's well-being. Although the family had given Allan more opportunities to interact with others, Allan had exhibited behaviors that were beginning to interrupt his activities. For example, Allan had decided to carry wipes in his pocket, and he would frequently clean doorknobs and play surfaces even when no food was present. He would also ask his teacher if he could wash his hands eight or ten times during the day, even though he had not eaten. At home, Allan asked questions about cleanliness and what his family members were eating. His family and I were concerned about these new behaviors Allan employed to avoid peanut in his environment.

Allan was concerned about cleanliness in general. He seemed to understand that casually touching a peanut would not likely cause him any significant ill health, but he was still particular about the cleanliness of his environment. Further probing revealed that his father, mother, and a sibling also displayed repetitive cleaning behavior and recurrent concerns and worries. Allan seemed to be experiencing a mental health disorder termed *obsessive-compulsive disorder,* which can run in families.

Although a certain level of concern about avoidance is necessary to promote safety, for Allan in two periods of his life, concern about avoidance had prevented him from normal involvement in day-to-day life activities and enjoyment. At this point, it was again affecting his state of general health and well-being. His previous exclusion from activities was based on his family's concerns about his allergy, which improved when the allergy was better understood. His new concerns were primarily a manifestation of a mental health disorder, separate from his food allergy but intertwined with it. Through counseling and medication, Allan was able to reduce these behaviors significantly and focus on school, friends, and a happy life.

Because diet restrictions are imposed, food allergy will to some extent affect day-to-day life activities. However, when food allergy results in overexclusion from life experiences, or causes a poor state of well-being, then the balance must be redirected. In many situations, a better understanding of your child's food allergy can help you and your child to ensure a happy and healthy lifestyle. However, if things become overwhelming, it is important to discuss these issues with your doctors and seek appropriate help from friends, family, other families sharing these types of experiences, clergy, or other support systems. If needed, seek help from psychologists, counselors, or psychiatrists. While your child may be suffering primarily from the consequences of food allergies, it is always important to remember others in the family, including siblings, parents, and, often, extended family. Making sure that everyone is included in the solution is the key to success. Lay organizations such as a the Food Allergy & Anaphylaxis Network and local support groups can help tremendously, and in the resources section of this book, you will see additional useful materials. Understanding you are not alone and that others have faced and solved similar problems can be a first step in getting the right help for your child and family.

PART 7

FOOD ALLERGY IN THE LONG TERM

The good news for many infants and children with food allergies is that many food allergies can be outgrown. Studies over the past several decades clearly document that food allergies to milk, eggs, wheat, or soy are primarily childhood problems. However, some of the more recent studies have shown both an increase in food allergy in general and also a parallel slowing of the rate of resolution in various food allergies. Studies in the past decade have shown an increase in allergies, not just to foods but also to other allergens, such as pollens, and an alarming rise in allergic disease such as asthma, atopic dermatitis, and hay fever. The possible cause for this recent increase in allergic disease, and the parallel increase in food allergies, has been explained by the hygiene hypothesis. *According to this theory, clean living has led our immune system to attack harmless proteins in the environment, like foods, pollens, or animal danders. The recent increase in allergies has led to an interest in preventing allergies.*

In Part 7, I explore the usual course of food allergies and how you and your allergist may work together to determine whether your child's food allergies are dissipating or persisting. I also consider the possible reasons for the recent rise in allergy in industrialized countries and what may be some of the risk factors for allergies. Finally, I discuss the various efforts to prevent allergies and food allergies through changes in diet.

28 ~ The Natural Course of Food Allergy

Marilyn is a 5-year-old with milk, egg, and peanut allergies, who I had followed since she was 1 year old. Her first reaction to milk occurred at 12 months, she reacted to eggs at 16 months. Allergy tests indicated a peanut allergy. As I followed Marilyn through the years, I explained to her family that there was a high likelihood she would outgrow her milk and egg allergies and possibly the peanut allergy. At this visit, they were eager to know whether her tests looked favorable for these possibilities.

Resolution of Food Allergies

On the basis of studies performed two decades ago, it has generally been quoted that 90 percent of children outgrow allergies to milk, egg, wheat, and soy by their third birthday. However, studies performed within the last decade appear to show a lower rate of resolution of allergies to milk and egg. More recent studies indicate that approximately 85 percent of children outgrow milk or egg allergy by age 5, although some studies unfortunately document lower rates of food allergy resolution. This lower rate for outgrowing food allergies seems to parallel a recent rise in the number of children with food allergies.

Allergies to foods such as peanut, tree nuts, fish, and shellfish were long thought to be permanent. The idea that an allergy to peanuts was permanent arose from studies of school-aged children who were monitored over about seven to fifteen years. None outgrew their peanut allergy. However, over the past ten years, studies clearly document that approximately 1 in 5 young children with a peanut allergy outgrows the peanut allergy by age 5. The previous studies focused on an older age group of peanut-allergic children who had apparently established a permanent allergy, whereas the younger children still appear to have an opportunity to outgrow their peanut allergy. No one has conducted extensive studies on the natural course of tree nut allergies or seafood allergies. However, one study showed that at least 9 percent of young children outgrew their tree nut allergy by school age. In several studies that my research group conducted, it appears that 2 percent to 5 percent of individuals outgrow fish or shellfish allergy. Not many studies have been conducted on the natural course of allergies to foods other than the ones already mentioned.

Unfortunately, it appears that the rate of outgrowing a food allergy is much slower after a child is 5 or 6 years old. For the 5 percent to 15 percent of children who have not outgrown their allergy by the time they are 5 years old, it seems that most will continue to hold onto their allergy at least for several more years. Not many long-term studies on the rate of outgrowing milk allergy beyond early school age have been conducted. In my clinical practice, I have seen children of all ages, including teenagers, overcome milk or egg allergy. Limited studies have been done on the number of adults who still have a milk allergy. However, it is possible to have milk allergy into adulthood, and this is probably also the case for several of the other usually short-lived food allergies, such as egg, soy, or wheat allergy.

We do not know what happens to the body when a child outgrows a food allergy. Persons who are outgrowing food allergy will often have declining levels of IgE antibodies. For example, skin tests may become smaller or blood tests may show declining food-specific IgE antibody levels. However, it is clear that children continue to have positive allergy tests even though they have outgrown the allergy and are able to tolerate the food with no symptoms.

A food allergy resolves gradually. When we perform oral food challenges on children we hope will tolerate a food, and they do not, we often see that in subsequent years, they are able to tolerate more of the food before a reaction occurs and then eventually are able to tolerate full servings of the food without reacting. Because the allergy tests often remain similar over that period of time, a number of factors seem to be responsible for their ability to tolerate the food, aside from what the tests may reflect. How the digestive system works or how the immune system responds to particular proteins may be factors. Theories about why a test may remain positive while a food is eventually tolerated are discussed in Chapter 30.

When an allergist follows a child over time, the food-specific IgE test results are monitored with the hope that the tests will show a decline (smaller skin tests and lower blood test scores). Often IgE levels will increase to a particular food very early in the course of food allergy. A child may have increasing sizes of skin tests or higher levels of IgE antibody to a particular food from age 1 to 3, and then we may see the skin test size level off for a while and then decline. Because the tests are interpreted both in the context of the child's age and clinical problems, the allergist is weighing the test results and history to decide whether a food allergy is being outgrown.

Food allergies not associated with IgE antibodies (described in Chapters 3 and 4) follow a somewhat different course of resolution than the IgE-antibody-mediated allergies. Infants with mucousy, bloody stools—proctocolitis syndrome—typically are able to tolerate milk products and do not have the bloody stools after age 1. Children with food-protein-induced enterocolitis syndrome can often tolerate a food a year or two after their last episode and usually do not have these problems after age 3. However, some children hold onto their enterocolitis syndrome even beyond age 5 or 6. Allergic eosinophilic gastroenteritis in infants sometimes appears to resolve. Allergic eosinophilic esophagitis, particularly in older children, may be more persistent because there are adults who have the same disease that they seem to have possibly developed during childhood. When a child has atopic dermatitis associated with a food allergy but does not have positive tests to the foods that trigger the disease, the food allergies are generally outgrown within the first few years of life.

Evaluations

For Marilyn, I had been following both her skin test sizes and food-specific IgE levels for several years. Her tests over the years are given in the following chart. Blood test results are in units called kIU/L (kilo International Units per liter) using a particular brand of test (the CAP System FEIA), while skin test sizes are shown in millimeters:

Age	*Peanut IgE*	*Milk IgE*	*Milk skin test*	*Egg IgE*	*Egg skin test*
1 yr	14	20	3 mm	2	6 mm
2 yr	15	35	5 mm	3	7 mm
3 yr	13	10	5 mm	3	7 mm
4 yr	14	5	3 mm	5	6 mm

Each time tests were performed, I reviewed her history of exposure to the foods and discussed with the family what her current risks of an allergic reaction might be. Each time we discussed whether it would be prudent to undertake an oral food challenge to see whether she would tolerate the foods. However, the family had been satisfied with Marilyn's diet and her lifestyle. Now, at age 5, her family was more concerned because she was attending school, and they wanted more information about her ability to eat the foods. Her milk and egg skin test had declined in size, although tests were still positive the year before her current evaluation. Her level of peanut antibody remained unchanged over the previous years at a level of 14 kIU/L, a range in which most children have reactions of an unpredictable severity to peanut.

During the current visit, I performed skin tests to milk, eggs, and peanut, and these test results were similar in size to the histamine control, which roughly would indicate a 50 percent chance of tolerating the food. The blood levels to milk and egg were both at a level of 2 kIU/L, the lowest they had ever been, which, for her age, indicated about a 50 percent risk for a reaction. Unfortunately, her peanut test continued to be 15 kIU/L. When test results decline, I can draw an imaginary line connecting the levels over the years and project at what point, assuming the decline remains similar from year to year, food challenges could be attempted.

Most families would like to undertake oral food challenges when a child has at least a 50 percent chance of tolerating a food. Of course, as discussed in Chapter 11, different families, different children, and different types of allergies may all lead to different decisions about when to perform these food challenges. Marilyn and her family were ready, and we undertook food challenges to milk and egg. She happily passed these food challenges and was ingesting those foods. But would she outgrow her peanut allergy? Because she still had a high risk of allergy to peanut, and because her test results did not seem to be changing very much, outgrowing the allergy in the next several years seemed unlikely. Test results would need to decline before I could surmise when she might outgrow the allergy. Once she was older it might be reasonable for Marilyn to undertake food challenges for peanut.

Recurrence

Marilyn's parents wondered whether Marilyn's allergies to milk or eggs would return. In general children do not redevelop a milk, egg, wheat, or soy allergy after they had tolerated meal-sized servings of the food during a food challenge. However, our research group was the first to describe the recurrence of peanut allergy in children who have tolerated peanuts during a food challenge. Our group's findings, and now reports from several other groups, indicate that in about 8 percent of children, peanut allergy recurred in those who had passed their oral food challenge of a meal-sized serving of peanut. So far, all of these children whose allergies recurred had one thing in common: they did not include peanut as a part of their diet after they passed their oral food challenge.

These children typically avoided peanuts for about a year after passing the food challenge for peanuts. When they later tried eating peanut products, they experienced reactions. Although they had positive allergy tests during the course of their peanut allergy, some of them had very low or even undetectable test results around the time of their food challenge, which they passed. However, when they were developing symptoms again, their test responses had also increased. This observation with peanut differs from milk, egg, wheat, or soy because these foods are common components of our daily diet, whereas peanuts could be avoided more easily. It appears that infrequent exposure to a particular food to which the person is allergy prone may not be good for the immune system and may stimulate an allergic immune response.

The recurrence of an allergy after a period of avoidance raises several questions. How often would a child need to eat a food to not become allergic to it again? No one has performed studies on this question, but it appears that for the children who have made peanut a regular part of their diet, the allergy had not recurred. Therefore, families who undertake oral food challenges should plan to make the food a regular part of the diet if the results indicate no allergic reaction. This same practice should apply to fish, shellfish, and tree nuts.

Another question raised by the observation of recurrence of a peanut allergy is that avoiding a food could backfire and result in an allergy. This issue is discussed in detail in Chapter 29.

If an individual has not eaten foods like peanut, nuts, or fish for months after they passed an oral food challenge, then they should be retested to be certain that it is still safe for them to eat these foods. Also because of our experiences with peanut allergy recurrence, families should continue to carry emergency medications for a year or two after the oral food challenge has been passed. Discontinue carrying the medication when the child has routinely tolerated the foods and has no other food allergies.

Adding Foods Back to the Diet after an Allergy Has Resolved

Of course, Marilyn's family was excited to learn that she would be able to enjoy milk and eggs. Many times, when a food allergy has been outgrown, fears remain about ingesting the once dangerous food. I tell the child that we have not seen any problem from the food and that it now seems safe for the child to include the food in her diet. Of course, when adding foods back to the diet, if there are still certain food allergies, care must be taken to avoid these allergens in products that are newly allowed in the diet. For example, Marilyn could now have ice cream but would need to be careful about peanut ingredients in the ice cream.

The good news for many children with food allergies is that allergy to milk, eggs, wheat, and soy typically resolve by age 5 years. Recent studies show that about 1 in 5 young children with a peanut allergy may no longer have that allergy by age 5 years. Although fewer people outgrow a tree nut or seafood allergy, some do. By following the clinical history and allergy test results, it is often possible to determine when a child may be outgrowing a food allergy and when a decision may be made to perform an oral food challenge. Recent studies have unfortunately shown that sometimes when an allergy has resolved, it could return, which has been noted for peanuts. It seems that once a child can tolerate a food, that food should eaten regularly to maintain the immune system's ability to ignore the food.

29 ~ Preventing Food Allergy

André and Marta were parents of a 3-year-old, highly allergic child. Their daughter had food allergies, asthma, and atopic dermatitis. Marta was six months pregnant and wanted to know what she could to do to help prevent allergies and food allergies in her soon-to-be-born child. Both Marta and André themselves had allergy problems such as asthma and, over their lifetime, eczema. Marta also had a food allergy to shellfish. Her daughter had peanut allergy. They wondered what the risks would be for their next child and how to reduce them.

Risk of Allergy

The allergic diseases, asthma, atopic dermatitis, hay fever, and food allergy, tend to run in families and occur in the same individuals. These are inherited disorders with a genetic component. Any person selected randomly from the general population may have a modest risk of having these allergic disorders. However, a child born to parents who both have allergic problems is more likely to have allergic problems than if the child had been born to parents without these problems. For Marta and André's soon-to-be-born infant, it was highly likely that allergic problems would arise, considering that all three of the family members had multiple allergic problems. Studies on specific risk factors are relatively few. It has been estimated that if both parents, or parent and child, have significant allergies, 70 percent to 80 percent of the time their next child would also have allergy problems. If only one parent has allergy problems, the risk drops to about 40 percent to 50 percent. The specific allergic problems family members experience are more likely to occur in the other family members. For example, if both parents have asthma, then there would be a high risk that the child would also have asthma.

We performed studies looking at siblings' risk for peanut allergy. If a sibling had a peanut allergy, which was the case for Marta and André, there is a 7 percent risk that another sibling would have this allergy as well. In addition, on the basis of Marta and André's family history, their newborn baby would likely have several allergic diseases, with unpredictable severity. It is never possible to predict exactly what to expect in any given child. I have seen many families where some of the children are suffering with multiple allergic problems and others have absolutely none. No tests can accurately predict which allergies a child may develop. People have tried to perform various tests on the blood of newborns, but the best "test" seems to be whether other members of the family have allergies.

The Rise in Allergies and Food Allergies

Marta and André knew that their family histories would indicate a higher risk that their children would have allergic problems. However, allergic problems in children and adults are on the rise. Environmental influences play a role in the recent rise in allergic disease. In the past two decades, asthma has doubled, atopic dermatitis has nearly tripled, and allergic rhinitis may also have doubled. We performed studies looking at the rate of peanut allergy in children in 1997 and again in 2002. Over that five-year period, the rate of peanut allergy in children increased from 1 in 250 children to 1 in 125. Similar results have been seen in other westernized countries such as in England.

Are we getting better at diagnosing more allergies now and talking more about allergies, or is there a true increase? Various studies indicate that our immune systems are attacking harmless proteins in the environment at a higher rate than ever before. In studies that performed allergy skin tests on the general population, without selection for people with specific allergic complaints, it has been documented that the number of positive tests has increased, more than doubled, within the past two decades. Because heredity does not change that quickly, environmental changes must be contributing to allergic disease.

Theories about the rise of food allergy abound: Perhaps dietary changes are responsible. For example, one theory suggests that roasted peanuts may be more allergenic than fried or boiled peanuts. In Asia, there is less peanut allergy, and children ingest fried or boiled peanut, whereas in the United States roasted peanuts are ingested. However, this theory is faulty because aside from peanut allergy, the allergy rate in general in Asia appears lower. Another theory is that mothers ingesting peanut and passing it into their breast milk may increase peanut allergy in babies who are ingesting peanut protein–laden breast milk. However, pollen allergy and cat allergy have also increased, and as far as I am aware, breast-feeding mothers are not eating more cats or tree pollen than they did in the past. Another food-specific theory to explain a rise in food allergy is that the use of antacid medications makes people more prone to a food allergy. The theory goes: acid in our stomach helps to digest proteins so our immune system does not see the protein in a form that is easier to recognize and "attack." While there is some evidence for this concern, it does not seem to explain the rise in allergy for asthma, hay fever, and atopic dermatitis. Therefore, we turn to our environment and consider how it may be turning our immune systems against otherwise harmless proteins. The primary theory to explain this increase is called the *hygiene hypothesis.*

The Hygiene Hypothesis

Hygiene, or cleanliness, may be a factor that has altered our immune system's response to our environment. Our immune system was designed to fight infections such as parasites or worms, viruses, and bacteria. The parts of the immune system that cause allergy are the same parts used to fight parasitic infections. However, westernized countries do not have a problem with parasites. Some maintain that a part of our immune system that would normally be fighting parasites is idle and attacks otherwise harmless proteins in foods or in the air, such as pollens. Another part of the cleanliness theory points to the various ways in which we have reduced the need for our immune system to fight infections to bacteria or viruses. For example, we will readily use antibiotics to fight bacterial infections, thereby making it easier on our immune systems. We also, as a community, receive vaccinations so that the number of illnesses or the degree of illness is reduced in our society. We are also somewhat fixated with cleanliness, washing our hands and keeping our homes clean, and so a variety of types of germs that may have otherwise kept our immune system busy are being removed from our environment.

What are some of the examples of evidence to support this hygiene hypothesis? It has been found that children who attended daycare centers had less asthma than those who did not. Presumably, exposure to the other children's germs was good for the immune system. It has also been observed that children born later into a family will less likely have allergies than those born earlier, again implying that exposure to older siblings' germs may have been protective in regard to allergy. Individuals growing up on farms with farm animals, with exposure to their manure and germs, also experience fewer allergies. Some studies have shown that allergies are less common in populations that have not been immunized as much or have experienced more natural infections such as tuberculosis or measles. Growing up with pets in the home has been associated with a reduced risk of allergy to those pets. Researchers believe the reduction in pet allergy for pet owners is associated with exposure to the germs from the animals.

Certain bacteria may be more protective than others in stimulating a "good" immune response to reduce the risk of allergy. Children born by Cesarean section seem to have a higher risk of allergy than those who are born vaginally. Exposure to the vaginal bacteria may help protect against allergy. In one study, the types of bacteria found in children who were allergic were different than the types of bacteria found in the feces of children who were less allergic.

To reduce or prevent allergy, no one is advocating ending vaccination, not using antibiotics, or reducing general hygiene. Individuals are living longer and healthier lives because of medications and vaccines. It is probably also quite impractical to have a farm animal living in your apartment as a means of allergy prevention!

Autoimmune diseases have also increased over the past several decades. Autoimmune diseases occur when the immune system attacks the body. Multiple sclerosis, rheumatoid arthritis, and lupus are autoimmune diseases. The rise in these disorders, and in allergy, indicate that our immune systems are attacking innocent proteins such as those in foods, pollen, and our own healthy cells.

Can a child's immune system be strengthened to avert allergies? In some sense, an allergic response is a strong but misdirected immune response. In fact, steroid medications commonly used to treat allergies are effective because they weaken or soften the immune response. The challenge for the future to turn off these allergic responses will likely require redirecting the immune system so it will remain strong but not attack harmless proteins in foods, pollens, or animal dander. One of the future goals for prevention of food allergy and other allergies may be to keep the immune system "busy" with treatments that promote healthy immune responses. In that way, we can have the best of both worlds: prevention of infection and of allergies.

Prevention of Allergy through Dietary Alterations

For over seventy years, studies have looked at the possible effect of diet in preventing allergic problems such as asthma, atopic dermatitis, hay fever, and food allergies. Preventing a medical problem can be looked at in several ways. True prevention could imply that something was done to forever stop the occurrence of an illness. However, prevention is often thought of as delaying or reducing an illness.

Let's look into our crystal ball. We see a child whose milk allergy will appear by age 1, and resolves by age 2. Therefore, if her parents had withheld milk until age 3, the milk allergy would never have been apparent. One could argue that the milk allergy had been *prevented.* If the parents had given the child milk at age 1½ and noticed a reaction, stopped the milk, reintroduced it at age 3 at which time the child tolerated the milk, they would have concluded that the child had *outgrown* the milk allergy. In the second situation, prevention would not have been considered. However, our crystal ball revealed that both situations actually had the same potential for allergy and resolution all along. Many studies in which a food is withheld from the diet suffer from this limitation; that is, one would not see an allergic response to a food the child never ingests. Does the long-term outcome change for that child by avoiding certain foods early in life?

A perfect study of food allergy prevention would require constant vigilance of every exposure; participants would be randomly assigned to test certain allergens. A perfect study is impractical and unethical because it is not possible to ask some families not to breast-feed and others to breast-feed. Because of these limitations, most of the studies on food allergy prevention are imperfect and must be interpreted with caution.

The first step in considering prevention measures is to determine who may best benefit from alterations in the diet. Most studies focus on high-risk families such as Marta and André. Unfortunately, some children are destined to develop allergies even without a family history of allergy. Nearly 50 percent of children who develop allergies do not have a strong family history of allergy. However, it is far more likely that a family with a history of allergy would have children with allergies and with more serious allergies. Therefore, most prevention measures have traditionally addressed families at high risk.

Diet in Pregnancy

Would dietary restrictions of particular foods during pregnancy alter the outcome of food allergy? Studies performed primarily outside of the United

States seem to indicate that dietary exclusion during pregnancy has no effect on outcomes for food allergies. A study from England showed that maternal ingestion of peanut during pregnancy did not have an effect on peanut allergy in children. One way scientists try to assemble information on a topic is to select the best studies and analyze them together as though examining one large group. This is called a *meta-analysis*. Meta-analysis of avoidance diets during pregnancy did not show a decrease in allergic diseases but did show that diet restrictions during pregnancy could affect the mother's or fetus's nutrition. Recommendations from various professional organizations around the globe vary slightly in regard to recommendations to families who may have a child at risk for allergic disease. In 2000, the American Academy of Pediatrics had recommended avoiding peanuts in the third trimester of pregnancy for families at risk of allergy, which was defined as a mother and child or both parents with allergies. This recommendation had been made on expert opinion but had not been thoroughly investigated to verify the impact. Since then, one study showed no influence in a mother's diet during pregnancy on a child's risk for peanut allergy.

Diet in Breast-Feeding

Alterations in the diet to prevent allergy could be undertaken while a mother is breast-feeding. We know that what the mother ingests may pass into breast milk, but does this exposure increase the risk of developing an allergy? A few good studies examine this question. In one study on peanut allergy, there was no association between the mothers' intake of peanut during breast-feeding and peanut allergy. In studies looking at multiple foods barred from the diet, there appears to be less atopic dermatitis in the first year or so of life but not a lasting effect. This raises the issue of whether food avoidance during breast-feeding is protective in the long run or just protective at a time when the child may have had problems from the food anyway. If only the latter is true, one could argue not to alter the diet unless an allergy-related illness was occurring.

In a study performed in the United States, where mothers eliminated highly allergenic foods from their diet while breast-feeding, compared with families where the mothers did not avoid these foods (for example, milk, egg, peanut, and fish), there was less milk allergy and less atopic dermatitis in that first year or two of life. But when the same children were followed to ages 4 and 7, there were equivalent numbers of children who had milk allergy, other food allergies, or atopic dermatitis. Therefore, no long-term prevention was achieved. To some extent, the jury is still out on whether maternal avoidance diets during breast-feeding have an effect on allergy outcomes. Some professional organizations, at some times, have recommended avoidance diets during breast-feeding for high-risk families like Marta and André, while others have not. Many breast-feeding mothers with other children with allergies avoid particular foods the other siblings cannot eat. These are often personal decisions. Marta was already not allowing peanut in the home, and so it seemed natural that she would avoid this food during pregnancy and breast-feeding, whether or not it truly had an effect on allergy outcomes.

Breast-Feeding for Prevention

Aside from the mother's diet while breast-feeding, does breast-feeding protect against allergy? Exclusively breast-feeding for the first four to six months of life is generally recommended by the American Academy of Pediatrics. Many studies have looked at the benefits of breast-feeding in general in effecting allergic disease. In a variety of meta-analyses on this topic, breast-feeding seems to have a protective effect compared with milk-based infant formulas, particularly among infants who are at high risk for allergy. Breast-feeding exclusively decreased the risk of atopic dermatitis by about one-third compared with feeding the cow's milk-based formula. Similarly, when numerous studies are analyzed together, there seems to be a protective effect of breast-feeding on asthma as well. This effect was primarily noted for families at high risk of having a child with allergies.

One European expert panel concluded that breast-feeding exclusively for at least four months in an allergy-prone infant is associated with a lower risk of milk allergy until at least age 18 months. Studies that have looked at the effect of breast-feeding on allergic outcomes have generally shown the strongest differences for allergy-prone families and have not generally looked long term, beyond the first several years of life. Occasional studies show counterproductive effects of breast-feeding in some allergy-prone infants. However, at this time, it seems that the preponderance of the evidence about breast-feeding is that it is generally protective against allergy, and breast-feeding is generally recommended exclusively for the first four to six months of an infant's life.

Solid Foods

What effect solid foods or additional foods in an infant's diet have on allergy has not been thoroughly investigated. One study evaluated allergy-prone families for whom mothers were asked to restrict allergenic foods from their diets during breast-feeding. Milk was not given to babies until age 1; egg was given at age 2; and peanuts, nuts, and fish at age 3. These children were compared with children from families that did not restrict these allergenic foods. In the first few years of life, less milk allergy was evident in the group on the diet, but by the ages 4 and 7, there was no significant difference in the number of positive skin tests or food allergies to the targeted foods. The study was limited because it did not monitor the diets, and many families dropped out of the study.

In a 2000 statement, the American Academy of Pediatrics recommended that families at high risk of their child having allergies consider avoiding these particular foods for the periods of time evaluated in the study. European groups and subsequently U.S. groups have indicated there is little evidence of long-term protective effects by doing so, admitting also that few studies have been conducted in this area to know for sure. For example, in Israel, peanut is generally included in the diet at a very early age, and not much peanut allergy exists there compared with the United States or England, where peanut is typically introduced later into the diet. One study showed an increased risk of allergic disease associated with delayed introduction of allergenic foods, such as eggs. These studies are sometimes difficult to interpret because families with allergy-prone children may purposefully avoid more highly allergenic foods until their children are older. Therefore, the study may look like avoiding the food caused the allergy, when, in fact, the presence of allergy caused the family to avoid the allergenic food.

Infant Formula

Numerous studies have looked at the role of infant formulas in causing or preventing allergies. The long-term effects of one formula or another remain unclear. Some studies indicate that a few milk formula feedings in the newborn nursery may increase an infant's likelihood of a milk allergy. Cow's milk–based formula is associated with an increased risk of atopic dermatitis and a milk allergy, at least during infancy, and very early childhood. Substitution with a soy-based formula does not seem to add a protective effect according to meta-analysis of various studies. One study suggested that using a soy formula may predispose infants to peanut allergy.

Extensively hydrolyzed, milk-based formulas are typically considered safe for a child with milk allergy. Recall that these are milk-based formulas in which the milk protein has been broken into very small pieces usually not

IN DEPTH ON WHAT MICE MAY TELL US ABOUT PREVENTION OF FOOD ALLERGY

The rise in allergy and food allergy has paralleled an increase in breast-feeding in the United States, but as indicated previously, all types of allergies have increased, and it is hard to assume that breast-feeding caused these allergies in the population. Both food and environmental allergens can be detected in breast milk. The body's immune system and digestive processes are designed so that the infant is exposed to the foods the mother ingests. This raises the possibility, at least theoretically, that there is a reason foods ingested by the mother are passed into breast milk and, therefore, the baby is exposed to these proteins. It is an unnatural consequence of our society that we feed the milk of cows to human infants or that we feed processed baby food to infants. One could otherwise surmise that solid foods would need to be given to infants at an older age, and one could argue a mother altering her diet to eliminate potential allergens is not natural and may prohibit the infant's immune system from "testing" the types of foods that she would eat later on. It is not so clear that this type of exposure would be counterproductive and exposure to maternally ingested foods through the breast milk could be helpful for the infant's immune system.

Although it seems to make sense that avoiding particular foods may allow the immune system to forget about these foods, studies on this topic are not so clear cut. For example, in research studies of mice, it is difficult for a mouse to develop a milk allergy if it has been raised on food that contains cow's milk. These mice, whose immune systems have been exposed to milk fairly regularly, are no longer likely to become allergic to this protein. To make an animal allergic to a food, it is usually necessary to exclude the food early on and then feed the food to the animal intermittently. Sometimes giving a very large dose to these mice or giving continuous small doses prevents the mouse from becoming allergic to the food. The type of exposure that is best at promoting an allergy in mice is to give intermittent bursts of exposures. If a family were avoiding food allergens in an infant's diet, then perhaps the immune system would have no reason to mount an attack to that food. However, even with strict avoidance, unavoidable, intermittent exposures could occur because food is a very common substance, and it may be impossible to exclude all exposure.

Avoiding the ingesting of a food allergen opens the possibility that the immune system will "see" the food through a route other than the mouth, an exposure that may be counterproductive. For example, mice prevented from eating a food allergen, such as eggs, can be made allergic to egg through repeated inhalation or skin exposures. In a study of peanut allergy risks in children in England, the development of a peanut allergy was associated with using topical skin creams that may contain peanut (which are not widely available or used in the United States). However, peanut allergy was not associated with the breast-feeding mothers' use of nipple creams that contain peanut, which the infants would have ingested. These observations could support the idea that widespread skin contact with peanut increased the risk for peanut allergy, while mouth exposure did not. This observation in humans is similar to what was described for mice, where allergy could be induced by repeated and extensive skin contact. If this is the case for humans, it seems reasonable to theorize that avoidance diets may be problematic if exposures are occurring anyway through intermittent skin contact, inhalation, or possibly ingestion. The theory that strict avoidance may be helpful to prevent or lose an allergy could be true, but the practical outcome may not work out for most individuals because complete avoidance may not be practical.

Another observation from studies of mice is that different strains require different doses of a food protein and different schedules of exposure to achieve or prevent allergies. Different strains of mice are similar to different individual humans. If humans are like the mice, it may well be that one child would be triggered to develop an allergy from a certain set of exposures, while another child might not. At this point in time, we do not have any way of knowing which child, if any, may benefit from a particular regimen of avoidance or exposure to a food to prevent an allergy to that food.

Mice studies also demonstrate how the environment relates to the development of allergy. Experimental studies show that it is easier to induce food allergies in mice treated with antibiotics early in their lives. This observation supports the "hygiene hypothesis" and the likely possibility that several aspects of the environment interact with various aspects of hereditary "risks" in regard to allergic problems.

Let us reconsider the recurrence of peanut allergy: children who ingested peanuts successfully during an oral food challenge avoided the food for nearly a year and then tried to eat peanut again but reacted. We could argue that it may have been better for them to continue to ingest the food that they tolerated. Like prevention, the recurrence of allergy demonstrates that exposure to a food may not be bad for the immune system in certain circumstances. I generally advise people to continue eating any food they already are eating and tolerating, even if, for some reason, they were tested positive to the food, just as persons who pass an oral food challenge, even with positive allergy tests, are instructed to eat the food they tolerate. I fear that if they stopped eating the food they tolerated, even with the positive test, they may have problems when they try to ingest the food at a later date.

When we consider all of these examples, it is less clear that avoidance diets would be helpful for preventing food allergies for everyone in every circumstance. In addition, we have recently focused on prevention or treatment of allergy through different means, for example, by stimulating good, nonallergic immune responses or exposing the immune system to the problem food in ways the immune system will accept food, not attack it. These treatment strategies, which are different than avoidance strategies, are the basis of future treatments of food allergies discussed in Part 8.

---

recognized by the immune system. In *partially hydrolyzed* formulas, milk protein is broken down but not as much. For a child who has a milk allergy, the partially hydrolyzed formula is likely to induce an allergic reaction. How useful are these formulas for preventing allergy in a child prone to a milk allergy? Studies show that certain extensive hydrolysate formulas are useful in preventing or delaying atopic dermatitis or milk allergies and that certain partially hydrolyzed formulas are almost as good as the extensive hydrolysates. Because the extensive hydrolysates lack taste and cost more than the partial hydrolysates, some experts recommend the partial hydrolysates as a prevention formula if breast-feeding cannot be continued and if cost and taste matter. However, whether these early interventions have long-term effect on allergies has not been proved. Amino acid–based formulas, which are not allergenic for individuals who may react to extensive hydrolysates, are costly and bitter tasting, and they have not been evaluated in studies of allergy prevention.

For Marta and André, breast-feeding for the first four to six months was the best start for good health and to avoid allergy. If their baby developed allergies, then the focus would switch from prevention to treatment. At that point, we'd consider whether to change certain foods or formulas. I did not recommend that Marta alter her diet during pregnancy. If she wanted to alter her diet during breast-feeding, that would be up to her. Solid foods should not be introduced until age 5 or 6 months, and specific foods to try would depend on how the baby was progressing. If Marta were unable to breast-feed or needed a supplemental formula, I suggested they not use a regular cow's milk–based or soy formula because these formulas are associated with atopic dermatitis or milk allergy.

The recent rise in allergic diseases including food allergy seems to be a consequence of our current environment. Although heredity plays a strong role in these allergic problems, our environment has contributed to the rise in allergies. Prevention strategies to reduce allergic disease, including food allergy, have primarily focused on alterations in the diet to avoid problem foods. While this seems to result in some short-term success for infants prone to allergy, the long-term effects of these strategies are unclear, and there are some theoretical concerns that they could be counterproductive. Prevention through exclusive breast-feeding for the first four to six months of an infant's life with a low-allergen formula supplement if breast-feeding is not possible, seems to be the best advice for allergy prevention. Whether maternal restriction diets or avoidance of particular foods in the infant affect allergy outcomes is unclear. Concepts about prevention and development of food allergy are changing, so talking to your allergist to go over the most recent recommendations and to individualize strategies for your child is important.

PART 8

LOOKING TOWARD THE FUTURE

In the 1970s, when comprehensive catalogs of research studies were initiated, there were generally fewer than one hundred research publications about food allergy each year. The number of research publications about food allergy tripled in the early 1990s, and after 2000, a thousand or more research studies are published each year on some aspect of food allergies. This exponential growth in research interest in food allergy probably reflects a response to the increasing prevalence of the disease. This is excellent news for children suffering with food allergies because countless researchers are now working to improve the quality of life for allergy sufferers, to determine better ways to diagnose a food allergy and, most importantly, to find better treatments for food allergies. It is the sincerest hope of researchers that more definitive diagnostic and treatment methods will be available in the not-too-distant future.

Some of the typical food allergy research questions include: How frequent are food allergies? What makes a person prone to food allergies? What makes a particular food cause allergies? What are some of the problems and symptoms that food allergies can cause? Can we find better diagnostic methods? What is the natural progression of food allergy and when can a food allergy be expected to resolve? What can I do to prevent a food allergy? And, how can we treat or cure food allergies? Throughout this book, many of these questions have been addressed and answered using research studies performed within the past few years. In the next two chapters,

I focus on research aimed at improved diagnosis and treatment of food allergy. I put in context some of the results from countless researchers working to improve life for persons with food allergy. The rapid advances in food allergy research will likely have practical consequences for diagnosis and treatment in the coming years. Regularly review Internet resources listed in Part 9 and discuss questions and concerns with your allergist.

Before proceeding, let me say a few words about research. Medical research is typically divided into three categories. Basic science research *is laboratory-based research using "test tubes" or sometimes experimentation with animals that have, or are made to have, food allergies. In these types of research studies, immune responses are tested and allergenic proteins are investigated in various ways. Basic science research studies do not directly involve people in the experimentation. However, in food allergy research, blood samples from people with and without food allergies are often used so that the immune responses can be tested.*

Clinical research *studies people directly. Some clinical research studies are considered observational studies. In observational studies, various features of living with food allergy and experiencing a food allergy are monitored to learn more about the allergies. For example, a group of children with peanut allergy may be followed over time to see whether they outgrow the allergies, what types of mistakes are made that lead to allergic reactions, and symptoms children experience in a variety of settings. Many of the results of these studies have been covered in this book. Epidemiology studies of people with food allergy seek to determine the number of people affected and the types of allergies they have. From these studies, we learn about the foods involved, the types of allergic reactions, and whether a recent increase in food allergies has occurred. Some clinical studies of allergy sufferers involve interventions. One such intervention could include administering a medication to see whether it affects the outcome of a food allergy.*

Translational research *connects basic science and clinical research. In translational research, lab discoveries are tested on people and the results are examined in the laboratory. For example, a blood test taken from an individual experiencing an allergic reaction may be used to determine what parts of a food protein are causing the reaction. This could lead to the creation of modified, altered food proteins that could be injected into that food-allergic person so that the immune system no longer attacks the food protein.*

Regulations ensure that research is performed in a safe and humane fashion. Clinical and translational research studies that involve people, including children, are monitored to ensure that the research questions are relevant and the studies are performed safely and with the least risk to participants. Moni-

toring is conducted at many levels to ensure safety. Institutions performing research typically have review boards that monitor research for safe procedures and high scientific quality. In some cases, additional groups monitor safety concerns before and during the actual studies. Depending on the type of research, additional oversight might be required.

Before individuals enter a research study, they are informed of all aspects of that study. Research participants will be told the purpose of the study and why they qualify to participate. Sometimes individuals are invited to participate in a study but may not qualify. Before the study begins, risks and benefits are explained. When children are involved, a parent or legal guardian must consent to the child's participation, and the child must also agree. Sometimes benefits to an individual or child are minimal, but there are societal benefits. If a discovery is made, it may benefit everyone with the food allergy, even the participating child.

Any known or suspected risks associated with a study will also be explained in detail. Before beginning a research study, a participant is typically asked to consent, often in writing, to participate in the research or to have their child participate. A research study can be declined and the child can continue to receive usual care instead. In addition, it is typically possible to withdraw from a study after it is under way. Participating in a research study may be time consuming. Occasionally, research participants may receive specific benefits, for example, the use of a study medication or treatment, or additional evaluations by the investigators. In some cases, a small payment is given for the time commitment. Most individuals participate in research projects for altruistic reasons: to help advance research in diagnosis and treatment of food allergies.

When research involves laboratory animals, such as mice, guinea pigs, or dogs, review boards and research procedures oversee the humane treatment of the animals and ensure that the research investigation warrants the use of the animals.

Funding for research studies comes from many sources. Private funding comes from individuals or organizations. Sometimes an individual will donate to an individual investigator or group of investigators with whom he or she is familiar to help advance research. Some not-for-profit organizations distribute funds for research purposes. These organizations include the American Academy of Allergy, Asthma and Immunology or the American College of Allergy, Asthma and Immunology. Most private organizations that have provided funding for food allergy research began as parents' organizations. For example, the New York–based Food Allergy Initiative has donated millions of dollars in research funding for food allergy research. A group of parents and grandparents interested in advancing research for food allergies that have affected their family members established this organization. The Food Allergy & Anaphylaxis Network and several other organizations have also provided a means for private individuals to donate money for food allergy research.

Government agencies are a major source of research funding. Primary among the government agencies that provide grant support for research is the National Institutes of Health (NIH). The National Institute of Allergy and Infectious Disease is the NIH branch that distributes allergy research money. These government agencies have earmarked millions of dollars in research funding of food allergy research. Typically, investigators apply for funds from the government, and applications are competitively evaluated for distribution of available funds.

Both private and government funding are typically directed toward research studies developed and initiated by individual researchers or groups of researchers. In some cases, specific themes are targeted, and researchers are asked to provide their ideas for how the specific problem should be researched and solved. A private organization, or the government, may see a research need, say, the identification of triggering proteins in a particular food. These agencies may invite researchers who believe that they are capable of determining the solution to these questions to apply for the grant money. The applications are evaluated competitively and the best plans selected for funding. In some cases, an investigator with a particular idea for a research project may apply to these agencies, requesting funds to undertake a research idea. The applications for funds to undertake research undergo a peer review process in which experts evaluate and critique the application.

In contrast to the procedures for funding investigator-directed projects in food allergy, industries such as pharmaceutical companies or, in some cases, food companies may fund studies associated with their product. For example, a pharmaceutical company may develop a treatment for food allergy and would take the idea to individual investigators to develop a research program that tests the treatment.

My colleague Dr. Xiu-Min Li is researching traditional Chinese medicine to treat food allergy. Dr. Li was trained in China and is familiar with herbal remedies used there. Although there were no specific herbal remedies for food allergy, some symptoms were treated with herbs, and Dr. Li developed research theories and questions, called hypotheses, *to evaluate how these herbal remedies may be used to treat food allergies. She wanted to evaluate these herbal remedies on the mice she made allergic to foods. This approach was highly exploratory and initially her requests for funding from the government were denied. This is not unusual. If theories are untested and possibly not likely to have a favorable outcome, peer reviewers may be reluctant to spend tax dollars on such a risky project. However, the Food Allergy Initiative, a private organization that had supported numerous research projects in food allergy, saw the merit in her approach and provided funding. With this funding, she was able to show successful treatment of food-allergic mice, and she was able to begin to look at why these treatments might work. With this information in hand and showing promise, she was able to convince NIH of the merit of her approaches, and she received further funding to conduct specific evaluations. Because of these opportunities, her therapy may eventually be used in clinical trials.*

Researchers share their discoveries in many ways. Researchers in food allergy and other disciplines share their research ideas and results at yearly meetings. This stimulates further work and further successes. When researchers have preliminary information or results that are nearly verified, they will often report the results in a short research summary called an abstract. The abstract is a brief review of the research work and is often presented at research meetings. At that point, external committees or peer review typically does not review the research information. However, when researchers are prepared to submit final results of their studies, these are submitted for publication in research journals. But first, experts in the area of that research review the research results anonymously. This process of peer review helps to ensure that the information being reported is the result of studies that were conducted in rigorous and reasonable ways.

Some research programs are undertaken with collaborators united through larger programs. One example is the Consortium on Food Allergy Research sponsored by the National Institute of Allergy and Infectious Diseases of NIH and headed by Hugh A. Sampson, M.D., at the Jaffe Food Allergy Institute at Mount Sinai. This government-sponsored program includes expert investigators in food allergy research from several major academic research centers in food allergy in the United States.

Researchers report their results when they are verified and ready to be shared with other scientists and the public. People outside the research field are sometimes concerned that researchers are secretive about their advances, and the public is concerned that perhaps researchers are not eager to find cures because then they would have nothing left to research! In fact, research is performed in an open environment, involving many individuals, so collusion is impossible. Researchers press forward with advances and report results as soon as possible. A single individual cannot perform meaningful research in isolation, so laboratories typically involve numerous individuals, each playing a role in the research project. The urgency to discover therapies that benefit people would never retard research advancements.

The media may report on research findings, but their radio or newspaper reports can be confusing. In this book, I have placed research advances in context.

However, newspaper or magazine articles may occasionally misconstrue research results. One example occurred a few years ago when a group of researchers showed how activated charcoal could bind up peanut protein in a test tube. This led to some news stories about how charcoal could cure peanut allergies. The researchers had actually used a medicinal charcoal (not charcoal briquettes) mixed with peanut in a test tube to show that it could bind up the peanut proteins. However, there were never any studies on people using this potential treatment, and the treatment has potential pitfalls, which were reviewed in Chapter 15.

In many circumstances, putting together the results of a variety of research studies performed by different investigators is necessary to understand how a particular problem in food allergy should be approached. For example, hundreds of research studies have been conducted on allergy prevention, many with different results because of the circumstances and situations of each study. Although some studies have different outcomes, they can be reviewed together to make better recommendations based on the preponderance of evidence. As new studies with improved methods emerge, it is possible to make even better decisions based on those results. This is not a quick process and requires understanding and interpretation by experts in the field.

A major stumbling block in interpreting research studies is cause and effect. For example, on a hot day, the pavement is hot, and there are more people who develop heat stroke. If you were to measure the temperature of the ground, you would find that the temperature of the ground correlates with the number of people who develop heat stroke. You might want to conclude that a hot ground causes heat stroke, but you would be wrong because you were perhaps ignoring the fact that the sun was beating down, making the individual and the ground hot. Sometimes, in research studies, observations are made that perhaps are not directly connected to the illness under investigation, such as food allergies. Sometimes you have to dig deeper.

30 ~ Research for Improved Diagnosis

The limitations of our current ability to diagnose a food allergy are evident. Allergy blood tests and skin tests typically are not definitive, and, in many cases, allergy diagnoses are highly dependent on the medical history and results of elimination diets and oral food challenges. Not having a simple definitive diagnostic test leads to uncertainty and anxiety. A definitive diagnosis may require an oral food challenge, which might cause an allergic reaction. However, research studies show promise for improvements in diagnostic tests for food allergy.

Improved Interpretation of Existing Tests

For many types of food allergies, particularly where ingestion of the food leads to sudden reactions, food-specific IgE antibodies that detect the food are formed by the immune system. Skin prick tests or scratch tests are able to detect these food-specific IgE antibodies, and blood tests are able to measure the amount of these proteins circulating in the bloodstream. The larger the allergy skin test size, or the higher the level of food-specific IgE antibody detected in the blood test, the more likely it is that this particular result reflects a true allergy to the food. In other words, a strong positive test indicates a higher risk that the food will cause an illness for your child. This concept was discussed in Part 2. Unfortunately, test results are not simple "yes" (your child has allergies) and "no" (your child does not have allergies). Even so, existing tests have been studied in ways that have allowed allergists to use the results to provide specific information about your child's allergy.

Researchers evaluate existing allergy tests by comparing the results to the outcome of oral food challenges in children. To interpret a test for beef allergy in children who may or may not have beef allergy, you might perform an allergy skin test to beef or a blood test to detect IgE to beef on one hundred children, who may have beef allergy. Each child would undergo an oral food challenge to beef to determine whether an allergic reaction would occur. The result for each child would be compared against the test result of the skin and blood tests. You would then know the percentage of children at each test score who had an allergic reaction (or not) from the beef. These results could be used as a guide for other children with allergies to beef and whether their results indicated tolerance or reaction to beef. This testing has been achieved for only a handful of foods, as discussed in Part 2. However, the information has been valuable to help guide parents and children on whether to ingest or avoid a food or whether to undergo an oral food challenge.

Test results vary from food to food and by age and circumstance of illness. Although it is important for researchers to continue to evaluate more foods in this manner to gain information about existing tests, a major thrust of current research is to modify tests to improve their accuracy, for example, to give a "yes/no" response instead of a "maybe" and to also enhance the tests to reflect the severity of an allergy and not just the chances of having a reaction to a particular food.

Modification of Existing Tests

The allergic response is directed toward the protein in foods, and all foods have some amount of protein. A food contains a collection of proteins, and each of these proteins is made up of amino acids. The immune system may recognize one or many of the proteins in a food as well as any number of areas on that particular protein. Researchers have found that the features of the food allergy may vary depending on which of the proteins, and where on the proteins, your child's immune system has recognized.

It is not that common to have an allergy to apples, but if a person is allergic to apples, the allergic reaction probably occurred after an initial reaction to birch pollen in the air, when the immune system created IgE antibodies to that pollen. The same IgE can now detect birch-pollen-looking proteins in apples. Many birch-pollen-related proteins in apples can be destroyed by heating or digesting them, hence this allergy is usually mild and consists of an itchy mouth rather than an anaphylactic reaction (see Chapter 4). However, on occasion individuals have a severe apple allergy. These individuals' immune response is often directed to a different protein in the same apple, which is not destroyed easily by heat or digestion. The first individual has what is usually a mild apple allergy and applesauce is tolerated; the second individual has a more severe apple allergy and also reacts to applesauce. This implies that a test may be possible to determine whether the immune system is attacking the less important birchlike protein or the more tenacious apple protein. Such a test could identify the severity of an apple allergy and may become available in the coming years.

In addition to evaluating the specific proteins to which the immune system has formed an attack, it is also possible to investigate the places on a particular protein that the immune system recognizes. Research studies have shown that the behavior of an allergy could depend on the locations on the proteins recognized by the immune system.

Studies of proteins that trigger immune responses have considered allergy to milk, peanuts, and eggs. Researchers have found that it may be possible to determine, based on the location of the protein the immune system is attacking, whether the allergy was currently present and the likelihood that the allergy would eventually resolve. For example, a child has a positive skin and blood test to egg. If the tests are indeterminate, we would not know whether that child on that day was going to react to eggs, and we perhaps would do an oral food challenge to find out. In addition, we would not know at that time how likely it would be for that child to lose the allergy in the coming years. Studies on the location of the protein under attack suggest there may be ways to learn more to answer these questions.

Proteins are made of chains of amino acids that are like beads on a baby's bracelet spelling out the protein's characteristics. It is possible in the laboratory to determine where on that chain of letters the immune system is recognizing the words or parts of words. The results of tests to determine where on the protein the immune system will attack were compared with food challenge results or studies of which children did or did not lose their allergy and the severity of allergic reactions. It turns out that there is some relationship of the test results to these important outcomes. Moving toward confirming these results and perhaps creating a commercialized version of this test is a major research goal; it may be possible to do a test on a 2-year-old child that would say that this particular child is likely to have an allergy but outgrow it in a few years, compared with a test result that may say otherwise.

You may be wondering why the pattern with which the immune system sees the protein could reflect a different outcome for a particular allergy. Proteins, although very, very tiny, are actually three-dimensional structures that may be recognized, in part, based on their shape. Let us consider again the baby's bracelet beads that spell out: THIS IS A MILK PROTEIN. If we took this baby's bracelet and squished it up in our hand into a particular shape, it may turn out that the word THIS is next to the word PROTEIN. Let us imagine that this is how the protein looks to the immune system when a skin test is done or when the protein enters the body when it is eaten but not yet digested. Now let's consider that digestion may pull the baby's bracelet out, stretching it so it looks more like a sentence. Even though the chain is the same and the beads are in line, the shape is different. If your immune system can see the chain when it is in its predigested shape but not when it is stretched out, things may be different (a transient allergy) than if your immune system can see the chain in any shape, even after digestion (a persistent allergy), as shown in this diagram:

Before digestion:

T-H-I-S-I-S-A-M-I

N-I-E-T-O-R-P-K-L

After digestion:

T-H-I-S-I-S-A-M-I-L-K-P-R-O-T-E-I-N

Although this is a simple example, proteins in these foods are numerous, with complex shapes, and there are many ways the immune system interacts with them. Nevertheless, picking apart the immune response seems to be possible and is likely to result in better tests in the future. My colleague Wayne Shreffler, M.D., Ph.D., has developed procedures to miniaturize these tests so they can be done, someday, with just a few drops of blood.

Tests of Blood Cells

Food allergies are not only the result of IgE antibodies. In some food allergies, other cells in the immune system recognize food proteins and release chemicals that result in illness. For example, T cells are a type of immune system cell that may recognize food proteins and for some persons release chemicals that create swelling and allergic inflammation in the gastrointestinal tract. Allergic disorders not associated, or only partly associated, with IgE antibodies are difficult to diagnose without oral food challenges. One way these allergies might be diagnosed more readily is by taking a blood sample that includes cells involved in these allergic reactions, placing the blood sample in a test tube, and adding the food proteins.

If the cell in the test tube recognizes the food protein in a way that can result in a food allergy, the cell may release detectable chemicals. These tests have been tried for several of the food allergies that affect the intestines and skin, with unsuccessful results. Investigators have sometimes found that specific chemicals are released by these cells that indicate an allergy is likely, or these cells may become stimulated by "seeing" the food protein and begin to multiply in the test tube. Researchers have also found that the cells may show particular proteins on their surfaces that help them to find their way to places in the body, such as the intestines or skin. Thus far, these research experiments have helped us to better understand how the immune system may see a food and result in a reaction in one place in the body versus another, but they are not precise enough for making good diagnostic decisions regarding food allergy outcomes. The hope is that someday this test would help determine whether a child has a food allergy that typical allergy skin tests would miss.

Atopy Patch Test

In Chapter 12, the skin patch test, which differs from the allergy prick skin test, was discussed. With the atopy patch test, food is placed on the skin, usually under a metal cup or patch, for a day or two; it is removed and the skin is checked over the following days for a rash. If a person is allergic, a rash may show up several days after the skin has been exposed. The atopy patch test may therefore reflect a slower allergic response not reflected by the tests for IgE antibodies. These slower responses are usually attributed to the T cells discussed in Chapter 1 and are the likely cause for food allergic responses in some children with atopic dermatitis when the skin tests are negative or in eosinophilic esophagitis or other intestinal disorders associated with negative tests for IgE antibodies (Chapter 4).

Early studies performed in Finland using this patch test procedure showed that children who had immediate reactions to milk were likely to have a positive immediate prick skin test to milk and less likely to have a positive patch test to milk. Children who had delayed skin reactions after ingesting milk, for example, with the delayed onset of eczema, were more likely to have a positive patch test to milk and less likely to have a positive prick skin test to milk. However, overlap of test results was also evident. Neither test was perfect.

Since that initial investigation, many studies have been conducted, mostly in Europe, on using the atopy patch test for diagnosing food allergies, particularly when the skin tests may not be relevant to the reaction. Many of the results of various studies have some of the same limitations discussed in this book regarding prick skin testing and the blood test for food-specific IgE antibodies. Specifically, some individuals have a positive test and have a delayed reaction to a food or the test is negative, but they still experience a reaction. As additional tests and research studies are reported, it will become easier to make final comments on the effectiveness of the patch testing for the determination of these delayed types of allergies.

Allergen Test Kits

It is important to know whether a food is free from allergens. Food companies may have cleaning procedures for removing allergens from equipment that comes into contact with multiple products, some of which may contain allergens. How will companies know whether the equipment is clean? Several companies have established tests to detect allergens in foods. Some tests work like a rapid pregnancy test. Some tests detect even the tiniest trace of the food. These tests are used increasingly by industry; home test kits may be next. These kits and tests need to undergo further research.

One problem is a very practical one. If I test a slice of a cake and it is free from peanut, will I be certain there is no peanut elsewhere in the cake? Unfortunately, the answer is "No." How tests are interpreted presents problems as well. The tests can be made to be sensitive; that is, they may be able to detect trace amounts of food protein. Although this sounds like a positive feature, it does raise a concern. Such a test might detect levels of protein that are actually harmless. Therefore, studies are needed to determine just how much food allergen is dangerous.

Research studies have allowed us to use existing tests for improved diagnosis of food allergy. Prick skin and blood tests for serum food-specific IgE antibodies can now be used to give more definitive information regarding current allergy, and, by following the test results over time, the allergist has a better idea when a child may be outgrowing an allergy and may be a candidate for an oral food challenge. Future tests, probably with improved skin and blood tests that use specific, relevant proteins or specific, relevant parts of proteins in the testing, are likely to advance our ability to determine who is currently allergic, who may outgrow a particular food allergy, and who may provide information about the severity of an allergy. Unfortunately, the most difficult type of food allergy to diagnose is where IgE antibodies are not centrally involved. To better diagnose these allergies, testing cells in test tubes and skin patch tests may help us predict outcomes.

31 ~ Research for Treatment and Cures

The primary therapy for food allergy has been avoidance of the food and treatment for an allergic reaction with emergency medications should an accidental exposure occur. This is a rather disappointing approach. The hope and goal of research for food allergy are to provide better treatments and a cure. Research efforts for treatment of food allergy fall into two broad categories. First, are therapies that would be useful for any type of food allergy, and second are therapies directed at treating an allergy to a particular food.

Food Allergy Treatments That Are Not Food Specific

Anti-IgE

Most food allergies are caused by the production of food-specific IgE antibodies. These IgE antibodies float through the bloodstream and attach themselves to allergy cells such as mast cells, or basophils (see Chapter 1). If it were possible to eliminate these antibodies, then most types of food allergies perhaps would not occur. One way to try to neutralize these antibodies is to capture them as they float around in the bloodstream. To do so, a protein has been engineered that looks a lot like an antibody that our body makes to fight infection, called the IgG antibody. However, this special IgG antibody has been engineered to attach to a small portion of IgE antibodies that are only detectable when the IgE is floating in the bloodstream, not when it is sitting on an allergy cell. The treatment was devised this way to avoid disturbing the IgE while it is still on the allergy cell because otherwise the cell could be triggered to release chemicals like histamine that cause the allergic symptoms. Instead, the treatment only grabs the IgE while it is floating harmlessly in the blood. The IgE antibodies pop off the allergy cells from time to time, and so this therapy attaches to them, keeps them from getting back onto the allergy cell, and gradually clears them.

This type of therapy was studied among adults with peanut allergy. The medication was injected at three different doses. Some individuals received blank, or placebo, treatments. The treatments were randomly assigned to participants who did not know whether they were being treated with the medication or placebo; they and the researchers did not know the dose. The participants underwent oral food challenges to peanut before and after the therapy. Even on the placebo treatment, individuals were able to tolerate more peanut than they were without treatment. Obviously, there is a subjective aspect in an allergic reaction. However, in a dose-responsive fashion, individuals who received higher doses of the anti-IgE antibody treatment were able to tolerate more peanut protein. On average, before treatment, they tolerated one-half of a peanut, and afterward they tolerated the equivalent of nine peanuts. The study focused on peanuts, but the therapy is not specific for peanuts because the injected anti-IgE antibodies capture IgE, whether it is IgE for milk, peanut, or even cat or tree pollen protein.

Although these study results are encouraging, 1 in 5 individuals had no improvement in the amount of peanut they could tolerate, even at the highest dose of treatment used in the study. The exact formulation of anti-IgE antibody used in the study is no longer being manufactured. Another type of anti-IgE antibody is going to be tested for treatment of food allergy and is also the type that is already approved for use in severe, allergic asthma. The hope is that this formulation may afford better protection for food allergy.

The therapy, if found to be successful, is not curative. In the first study, the therapy was able to raise the amount of peanut the person could tolerate in most, but not all, of the participants. Still, reactions occurred once a higher dose was reached. This treatment may provide a margin of safety in the event of an accidental ingestion. If it turns out that this treatment is helpful, then an individual would need to remain on the therapy to continue to be protected. The first study showed that some people had no protection, so before using the therapy it would be necessary to know who may or may not be protected or what can be done to improve the treatment. If your child were on the therapy for severe asthma, it would be premature and possibly dangerous to expect the therapy to protect against food allergy until the studies are able to address the remaining questions about this therapy.

Traditional Chinese Medicine

As briefly reviewed in the introduction to Part 8, a concoction of herbs has been used to treat food-allergic mice. This concoction of herbs contained many ingredients and chemicals. Studies are trying to determine which of the ingredients is most active in treating food allergy. Studies using a limited number of the most active components researched in the animal models hopefully will be helpful for humans, and the plan is to perform studies to determine whether this treatment can reduce, cure, or perhaps prevent food allergies.

Probiotics

One theory about why food allergy is on the rise is that we are living in a relatively sterile environment, and bacteria that might promote a healthy immune response are not stimulating our immune systems. One approach is to provide "good bacteria" that may stimulate a protective immune response. Probiotics are a kind of bacteria that we may naturally find in the intestine that can be given, perhaps, to newborn infants, children, or pregnant or nursing mothers to try to establish a more healthy immune response. This treatment has been associated with some improvement in atopic dermatitis, although in children studied thus far, no improvement in food allergy was detected, and no difference was reported in allergy test results whether treatment was instituted with the probiotic. Many types of bacteria are used as probiotics, and some studies are now indicating that the type of bacteria may influence outcomes. Although these probiotics are typically considered safe, there are two cautions. First, some of them are derived from bacteria grown in milk, which could be an issue for individuals with milk allergy, and some individuals with a weak immune system acquired a serious infection from live bacteria.

Engineered Molecules That Turn Off the Immune System Responses

Similar to the engineering of IgG antibodies able to capture human IgE antibodies, injectable IgG antibodies engineered to neutralize chemicals involved in allergic responses or to block various allergic responses are being studied. The immune system produces several proteins that cause eosinophils to collect in the esophagus. These proteins have been identified as a possible target for treatment of eosinophilic esophagitis (described in Chapter 4). Injection of IgG antibodies engineered to capture the protein involved in this type of allergic inflammation may be able to reduce inflammation and provide relief for individuals with this allergy. Hundreds of molecules are involved in various allergic immunologic responses, and it may be possible to create specific treatments that target each of these molecules, to neutralize them, and to provide relief from allergic inflammation. Preliminary studies show promise, in particular for people with eosinophilic intestinal disorders.

Treatments for Anaphylaxis

Numerous chemicals are released from allergy cells during anaphylaxis. Research is under way to create therapies that may block the release of these molecules in the first place or interrupt the adverse responses they cause. For the immediate future, epinephrine remains the most important treatment for anaphylaxis. Improvements in epinephrine may be forthcoming. Research is under way to investigate the possibility of creating a form of epinephrine that can be given under the tongue instead of by injection. In addition, allergists are hopeful that additional doses of self-injectors of epinephrine will become available for infants.

Food-Specific Treatments

Conventional Allergy Shots

Allergy "shots" or, more specifically, immunotherapy, have been used for decades to treat environmental allergies, such as pollens that cause hay fever. An individual is injected with the same protein that causes the symptoms. Imagine a person who is allergic to pollen from a birch tree. When that birch tree pollen enters the eyes and nose, itching, sneezing, and nasal congestion occur. That person's immune system has learned to produce IgE antibodies to the birch pollen protein. The typical way that the person's body has identified the birch pollen is through interactions with the immune system at the surfaces of the respiratory tract, the nose, and the lungs. These are the same surfaces that often first contact parasites, an uncommon germ in industrialized areas. Many of the same immune processes in allergy are similar to those that fight parasite infections. What would happen if we suddenly changed the circumstance for our immune system and injected the birch pollen protein into the arm? Now a whole different part of the immune system would see that protein. The part of the immune system that attacks bacteria that may enter the body, for example, if you step on a dirty nail, will see the injected birch pollen in a new way. Instead of treating the birch pollen like a parasite, the immune system will treat it like bacteria; the allergic symptoms may fade when the birch pollen blows into the nose and lungs during pollen season. This strategy of injecting a protein to change the immune response has been used for foods as well.

Studies have been performed with individuals with severe peanut allergy wherein extracts of peanut are injected into the arm. Unfortunately, severe allergic reactions resulted from the injection of peanut in these individuals. However, during the study, it was also observed that individuals were able to tolerate, during doctor-supervised oral food challenges, a larger amount of peanut protein than without the injections. Therefore, researchers concluded that the injections worked but caused too many side effects to be practical, and the approach was abandoned. Injecting food proteins to treat allergy may be reevaluated if injections are combined with anti-IgE, which may reduce side effects from the injections.

Although injecting food protein has not met with success because of the side effects, the success that pollen injections has achieved for hay fever bodes well for treating pollen-related food allergy or oral allergy syndrome (see Chapter 4). Some studies show that when an individual undergoes allergy immunotherapy using the problematic pollen related to the food allergen, the food allergy declines. For example, a person with a birch pollen allergy who experiences an itchy mouth from eating peaches and apples may tolerate those fruits as the pollen allergy is treated. Study results have been mixed. In some individuals, the pollen-related food allergy worsened when this therapy was used. Whether a person should receive pollen allergy shots to primarily treat food allergy is debatable, and a doctor's guidance is recommended. However, if your child has hay fever symptoms and, as a result, qualifies for allergy shots for a food-related pollen, a potential good outcome may be the ability to tolerate the related foods. Candidates for pollen immunotherapy are typically individuals whose nose sprays and antihistamines for pollen allergy have not worked and whose symptoms persist despite these medications.

Oral Immunotherapy

Injection therapy with peanut protein showed promise but caused severe side effects. Another way to acclimate the immune system to an allergen may be by mouth. This treatment has also been used for pollens, with some success, and has been tried for food allergy. In some studies, food allergens have been given to food-allergic children or adults, starting with small amounts swallowed and gradually increased, over days, weeks, and months, although some studies have tried much quicker treatment times. The results have been promising but mixed. Most of the individuals in one study were able to tolerate the food after the procedure, and in other studies only some were able to. Some studies show significant side effects while the therapy was being undertaken that required some participants to stop. Sometimes it took a while to tolerate meal-sized portions of the foods; in those cases, the procedure may not have changed anything and the child simply outgrew the allergy. Some studies that showed success noted that a permanent tolerance of the food was not achieved, and the allergy recurred after a period when the food was not ingested. Some studies have attempted these treatments using small amounts of the food placed under the tongue, also with mixed results.

Ideally, studies should include blind, placebo, and randomized treatments and a control group treated with a substance that resembles the true treatment. This study, called a *randomized, controlled trial,* has not been reported thus far for this type of therapy. Because the results have been mixed and the procedure is potentially dangerous, it is still considered investigational and has not been widely adapted. However, oral treatment of allergies is potentially effective and remains a crucial area of study. In addition, ingesting allergens early in life as a way to prevent allergies is another area of active research.

Modified Allergens for Immunotherapy

Injecting food allergens may trigger allergic reactions. Therefore, researchers have focused on engineering, or creating in the laboratory, proteins that are similar to the food proteins but altered to prevent an allergic reaction when injected. Imagine taking a peanut protein that is able to cause anaphylaxis in an individual and changing that protein in a way that removes some or all of the places that an IgE antibody might attach. Now the remaining peanut protein still has many of the same parts as an unmodified peanut protein but is missing the parts that would trigger anaphylaxis. If this protein were injected, it might still be able to stimulate many parts of the immune system that recognize peanut protein but would not activate the allergy mast cells. Repeated injection of this modified protein could teach the immune system to "accept" peanut proteins (or whatever food is engineered for this use). Modified immunotherapy has shown success in animal models of peanut allergy. A similar approach involves an injection made by breaking up a food protein into smaller pieces less likely to trigger an immediate allergic response but still large enough to stimulate a good immune response that will no longer result in allergy.

Our immune system has learned to identify some molecules in a way that stimulates a nonallergic immune response. For example, molecules in bacteria generally lead the immune system toward a nonallergic immune response against the proteins in the bacteria. Allergy immunotherapy could be enhanced to include bacteria molecules that stimulate a good immune response. This therapy has been undertaken with some success in animal models of food allergy. Researchers create the altered, engineered food proteins by having bacteria produce these molecules. Therefore, the bacteria and the protein are left mixed together to create a food allergy treatment. This treatment has shown success in various animal models of food allergy. A similar approach that shows promise is to attach these bacterial molecules to engineered (modified) allergens for injection. One day it may be possible to mix proteins and molecules to stimulate the right immune response administered by injection, by mouth, or as rectal suppositories.

Another method for treatment could include attaching food allergens to molecules that attach to specific proteins on the surface of allergy cells, such as mast cells, that turn off those mast cells. In this type of therapy, the food protein may attach to an IgE antibody on a mast cell while, at the same time, the engineered protein attached to the food will tell the allergy cell not to release its histamine.

A variety of therapies in the pipeline attempt to reduce, treat, cure, or prevent food allergies. Anti-IgE promises to provide a safety net for individuals, whatever they are allergic to, but more studies are needed to ensure that this therapy is useful and to know how much protection an individual may have. Studies are evaluating how ingested or injected treatments with whole or modified food proteins may be able to alter the immune responses. In addition, treatment with probiotics and traditional Chinese medications may allow for improved therapy of food allergy. When a better treatment or cure for food allergy may be available is hard to predict. However, numerous studies are ongoing, with many promising results in animal models and treatment studies planned for human participants.

PART 9

KEEPING CURRENT

32 ~ An Action Plan for Anaphylaxis

On the following pages is one example of a written action plan for food allergy and anaphylaxis. The plan also shows how to use self-injectable epinephrine. *Notice that fingers are kept away from the ends of the unit and the injection is given into the front, outer edge of the thigh.* The plan is reproduced with kind permission from the Food Allergy & Anaphylaxis Network (www.foodallergy.org). You can download the latest version of this plan from its Web site.

Food Allergy Action Plan

Student's Name:____________________ **D.O.B:**__________ **Teacher:**________________	Place Child's Picture Here

ALLERGY TO:____

Asthmatic Yes* ☐ No ☐ *Higher risk for severe reaction

◆ STEP 1: TREATMENT ◆

Symptoms:		**Give Checked Medication****: (To be determined by physician authorizing treatment)	
▪ If a food allergen has been ingested, but *no symptoms*:		☐ Epinephrine	☐ Antihistamine
▪ Mouth	Itching, tingling, or swelling of lips, tongue, mouth	☐ Epinephrine	☐ Antihistamine
▪ Skin	Hives, itchy rash, swelling of the face or extremities	☐ Epinephrine	☐ Antihistamine
▪ Gut	Nausea, abdominal cramps, vomiting, diarrhea	☐ Epinephrine	☐ Antihistamine
▪ Throat†	Tightening of throat, hoarseness, hacking cough	☐ Epinephrine	☐ Antihistamine
▪ Lung†	Shortness of breath, repetitive coughing, wheezing	☐ Epinephrine	☐ Antihistamine
▪ Heart†	Thready pulse, low blood pressure, fainting, pale, blueness	☐ Epinephrine	☐ Antihistamine
▪ Other†	____________________	☐ Epinephrine	☐ Antihistamine
▪ If reaction is progressing (several of the above areas affected), give		☐ Epinephrine	☐ Antihistamine

The severity of symptoms can quickly change. †Potentially life-threatening.

DOSAGE

Epinephrine: inject intramuscularly (circle one) EpiPen® EpiPen® Jr. Twinject™ 0.3 mg Twinject™ 0.15 mg (see reverse side for instructions)

Antihistamine: give____
medication/dose/route

Other: give____
medication/dose/route

◆ STEP 2: EMERGENCY CALLS ◆

1. Call 911 (or Rescue Squad: ____________________). State that an allergic reaction has been treated, and additional epinephrine may be needed.

2. Dr. ________________________ at ________________________

3. Emergency contacts:

Name/Relationship	Phone Number(s)	
a. ____________________	1.)________________	2.) ________________
b. ____________________	1.)________________	2.) ________________
c. ____________________	1.)________________	2.) ________________

EVEN IF PARENT/GUARDIAN CANNOT BE REACHED, DO NOT HESITATE TO MEDICATE OR TAKE CHILD TO MEDICAL FACILITY!

Parent/Guardian Signature______________________________ Date____________

Doctor's Signature______________________________ Date____________
(Required)

TRAINED STAFF MEMBERS

1. ______________________________ Room ________

2. ______________________________ Room ________

3. ______________________________ Room ________

EpiPen® and EpiPen® Jr. Directions

- **Pull off gray activation cap.**

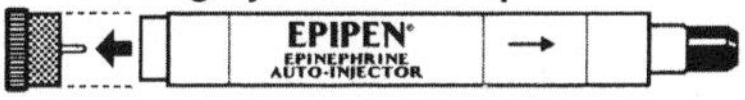

- **Hold black tip near outer thigh (always apply to thigh).**

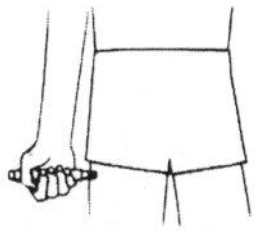

- **Swing and jab firmly into outer thigh until Auto-Injector mechanism functions. Hold in place and count to 10. Remove the EpiPen® unit and massage the injection area for 10 seconds.**

Twinject™ 0.3 mg and Twinject™ 0.15 mg Directions

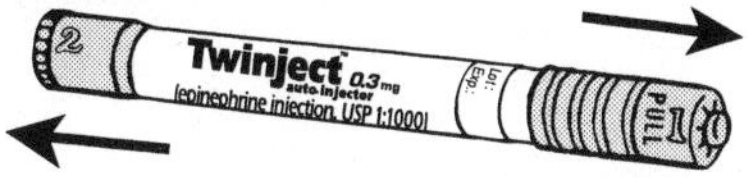

- **Pull off green end cap, then red end cap.**

- **Put gray cap against outer thigh, press down firmly until needle penetrates. Hold for 10 seconds, then remove.**

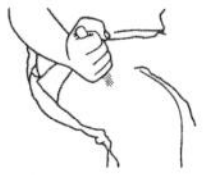

<u>SECOND DOSE ADMINISTRATION</u>:
If symptoms don't improve after 10 minutes, administer second dose:

- **Unscrew gray cap and pull syringe from barrel by holding blue collar at needle base.**
- **Slide yellow or orange collar off plunger.**

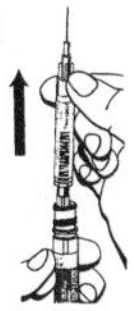

- **Put needle into thigh through skin, push plunger down all the way, and remove.**

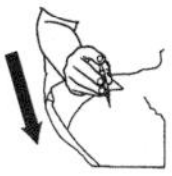

Once EpiPen® or Twinject™ is used, call the Rescue Squad. Take the used unit with you to the Emergency Room. Plan to stay for observation at the Emergency Room for at least 4 hours.

For children with multiple food allergies, consider providing separate Action Plans for different foods.

The Food Allergy & Anaphylaxis Network

***Medication checklist adapted from the Authorization of Emergency Treatment form developed by the Mount Sinai School of Medicine. Used with permission.*

33 ~ Food Allergy Resources

Although this book contains the most recent information about food allergy available at this writing, it is a wonderful consequence of the rapid rise in research that certain information may become "dated" or revised by new research. This is why it is vital that you discuss all diagnostic, treatment, and prevention matters with your doctor to ensure you are doing what is best for your child. In addition, increasing numbers of reliable sources for up-to-date information about food allergy are available.

There are also increasing resources with all types of important information and materials for families with children with food allergy. Resources include Internet sites, organizations with broad or specific interests, books about food allergy, food allergy cookbooks, books for children, companies that cater to producing specific allergen-free products, and companies that produce specialty items such as carrying cases for medications. Web sites abound with food allergy information. It would be impractical to list all of the resources. Internet information is not definitive, so peruse with caution. A few helpful sites are listed and will serve as gateways to many, if not all, of the resources mentioned in this book.

Nonprofit Resources

THE FOOD ALLERGY & ANAPHYLAXIS NETWORK (800-929-4040)
www.foodallergy.org

FAAN is a major resource for individuals and families with food allergies. The organization has an internationally recognized medical advisory board that oversees its materials. FAAN provides parent educational conferences; educational books and videos for parents covering most topics on managing food allergy; comprehensive programs for preschools, schools, and camps; books for children and teens; research updates; and much more. FAAN is also active in education, research, and policy regarding food allergy. The site is an excellent resource for current research and policies regarding food allergy. A newsletter is offered as well. A Web site and newsletter for children and teens are also offered.

FOOD ALLERGY INITIATIVE
www.foodallergyinitiative.org

This organization's mission includes raising funds to support food allergy research efforts, to raise public awareness about food allergy, and to improve safety for people with food allergies through education and public policy. The Web site provides excellent information on research in food allergy.

THE JAFFE FOOD ALLERGY INSTITUTE AT MOUNT SINAI
www.mssm.edu/jaffe_food_allergy

The Web site includes ongoing work at the Institute.

AMERICAN ACADEMY OF ALLERGY, ASTHMA AND IMMUNOLOGY
www.aaaai.org

AMERICAN COLLEGE OF ALLERGY, ASTHMA AND IMMUNOLOGY
www.acaai.org

These professional organizations have public information resources for allergy and food allergy. In addition, they offer search engines to locate board-certified allergists by entering your zip code and specific interests.

ASTHMA AND ALLERGY FOUNDATION OF AMERICA
www.aafa.org

This organization offers resources for people with allergic problems.

AMERICAN ACADEMY OF PEDIATRICS
www.aap.org

This is the professional organization for U.S. pediatricians. The site includes information for parents on a variety of health topics, including allergy.

MEDIC ALERT
www.medicalert.org

This nonprofit organization offers "linking" the medical identification jewelry to additional medical information. Several competing companies make medical identification jewelry.

AMERICAN DIETETIC ASSOCIATION
www.eatright.org

This is an organization of registered dietitians; the search engine can locate registered dietitians.

CENTER FOR FOOD SAFETY AND APPLIED NUTRITION
www.cfsan.fda.gov

This division of the U.S. Food and Drug Administration assists with matters of public health and policy regarding food safety, including allergy. Information about labeling and other food allergy issues are posted on this site. Report problems with foods (for example, undeclared allergen) through www.fda.gov/medwatch/.

For-Profit Resources

DEY PHARMACEUTICAL COMPANY
www.epipen.com

This Web site has helpful information about anaphylaxis, including a video showing how to use the EpiPen, the product this company distributes.

VERUS PHARMACEUTICAL COMPANY
www.twinject.com

This Web site has helpful information about anaphylaxis, including a video showing how to use the Twinject, the product this company distributes.

Glossary of Common Allergic Disorders

The allergic disorders listed below are described in this book. Here, additional brief information is provided for easy reference.

Most children with food allergy experience respiratory allergies. Some also have asthma or hay fever. These illnesses often develop in early childhood during a time when food allergies and atopic dermatitis may be improving. Insect sting allergy and drug allergy are only slightly more prevalent in children with food allergies than children without food allergies.

Allergic Rhinitis (Hay Fever)

Allergic rhinitis, or hay fever, which may also be associated with allergic eye symptoms called *allergic conjunctivitis,* typically occurs from an exposure of the nose and eyes to allergens in the air. The symptoms can include itchiness and redness of the eyes and perhaps some swelling, itchiness, and nasal congestion, often with a clear drip from the nose, and sneezing. A child may scratch or rub his nose. Often the rubbing follows a pattern called an *allergic salute.* Sometimes the child will rub his hand back and forth across the nose using the index finger; sometimes the child will use the entire hand from the tip of the middle finger to the bottom of the palm to swipe his nose.

It may be difficult to know whether your child's nose or eye symptoms are caused by a viral infection or an allergy, but usually with an allergy, the symptoms are related to seasonal exposures, such as pollen, or as the result of an exposure to animal dander. Allergy involves a lot of sneezing and itching; with viral, or cold, symptoms, thick nasal discharge occurs. Antihistamine treats the itch and sneezing. If there is a lot of nasal congestion, then a steroid nasal spray is often used to reduce the swelling and inflammation. These nasal sprays may take a few days to achieve maximal relief. They are not habit-forming like some of the over-the-counter nose sprays that give instant relief of nasal congestion. Sometimes medications that block specific pathways of allergic inflammation, such as antileukotriene medications, are also used. Additional treatments include decongestant medications, saltwater or moisturizing nose sprays, and other medicated sprays with antiallergy ingredients. Because allergy is the primary trigger in these symptoms, your physician will ask what triggers these reactions, or what time of year these symptoms occur. Allergy tests may identify the triggers. If there is not a good response to the various medications used to treat these symptoms, injections of the allergen, called *allergen immunotherapy* or allergy shots, may be used to quell symptoms. The specific allergens that may play a role in allergic rhinitis or hay fever will be described under "Environmental Allergens."

Asthma

Asthma is a common childhood disorder; it is more common in children who have allergic problems than in children who do not. Asthma symptoms include coughing and wheezing. A significant episode would also include shortness of breath, difficulty with air going out of the lungs, increased rate of breathing, or retractions, when the chest is pulling in during breathing. The nose may flare with each breath, like a rabbit's, if breathing trouble intensifies. Asthma is an inherited disease so it runs in families and accompanies the other allergic diseases described in this book. A viral infection, such as a cold, which causes increased mucus in the breathing tubes, can trigger an asthmatic reaction, or attack. Other triggers include exercise and cold air. Inhaled allergens can trigger or contribute to asthma.

Two main problems occur with asthma. The lungs are made of many, many tubes that carry air as we breathe in and out. The inside of these tubes is lined with a thin skin, and for people with asthma, this skin lining can swell and produce mucus. The swelling blocks the space air travels through and if mucus is produced air is further inhibited. A circle of muscle on the outer edges of the tube can become twitchy, causing the tube to close up. This constriction makes it harder to breathe through the already swollen and mucous-laden tubes. During an asthma episode, wheezing noises can be heard as air is forced through the narrowed tubes.

The doctor can hear the wheezing noises through a stethoscope, but you may observe your child's cough or labored breathing. Some asthma medications act immediately to stop the muscles from twitching, thereby opening up the tubes and allowing the air to go through. These medications are called *bronchodilators* and are rescue medications for asthma. Medications that help to reduce swelling and mucus come in many forms. *Cromolyn* helps to relax some of the allergy cells, called *mast cells,* in the airway. *Antileukotrienes* block certain reaction pathways that cause inflammation. Steroids are the strongest medications that help to reduce the swelling, mucus, or inflammation that may occur in the airways. Steroids may be taken orally in pill or liquid form and will travel throughout the body to reduce inflammation in the lungs. More commonly, physicians may prescribe inhalers (canisters or nebulizers) in which the inhaled steroids coat the airway and, therefore, work directly on the lungs to reduce inflammation. And the worrisome side effects of oral steroids, such as increased blood pressure or growth delay, are, therefore, avoided.

Although some parents are concerned about growth delay even from inhaled steroids, studies typically show that if used at their usual dosage over long periods of time, though there may be some initial slowing of growth, typically there are no long-term growth suppressive effects. Discuss your child's asthma in detail with your doctor to determine how best to monitor and to treat your child's symptoms. The types of medications selected and when and how they will be used are tailored to the severity of your child's asthma. Medications may change frequently over time as the asthma responds to various seasonal issues, exercise, or infections.

With allergic asthma, reducing the inhalation of items your child may be allergic to is crucial. For example, the swelling and mucus inside of the lung tubes can result from hard-to-avoid viral infections, but they can also result from an inhalation of allergens that may be avoidable. These environmental allergens will be discussed later in this section, but some simple measures to try to avoid them may go a long way for treating asthma. Irritants such as cigarette smoke should also be avoided.

Atopic Dermatitis

Atopic dermatitis is a type of eczema skin rash that typically occurs in individuals who have other allergic problems. Atopic dermatitis is described in detail in Chapter 3. This rash often develops during infancy and may persist through early childhood and sometimes into adulthood, but the character of the rash often changes with age. The primary features of atopic dermatitis are the extreme itchiness of the rash and that the rash affects certain typical areas of the body. In infants the rash often occurs on the outer edges of the cheeks, arms, legs, and, sometimes, chest and back. Often the diaper area is spared because there is not a lot of scratching that can occur there. Indeed, atopic dermatitis is often called "the itch that rashes" because scratching the itchy skin increases the rash. As children grow up, the rash tends to move behind the knees, in the elbow creases, around the neck, and in other creases of the body. The skin can become cracked, chapped, and open; infection can set in. Dry skin is a primary feature of atopic dermatitis. Sometimes the skin will thicken and extra creases will appear in the skin, particularly around the eyes or on the palms. Atopic dermatitis is an inherited disorder and often accompanies other allergic problems. The rash typically worsens, then improves over time, following an up and down course. A variety of nonallergic and allergic triggers of atopic dermatitis are discussed in Chapter 3, along with suggested treatments.

Drug Allergies

Allergies to medications can be caused by the chemical in the medication or sometimes the preservative or stabilizer ingredients. Tests that detect drug allergies are limited. If your child has experienced a possible allergic reaction to a medication, an allergist will often perform tests. But it is not usual to test before a problem develops. Discuss with your doctor the details of the symptoms you have observed in association with the medication. Like foods, drugs can induce varied reactions that may not be allergenic but may look like an allergy.

Environmental Allergens

Airborne environmental allergens fall into one of two categories: the indoor environmental allergens and the outdoor environmental allergens. Children with food allergies may also be sensitive to these common environmental allergens, which can contribute to skin and respiratory problems. The following list describes some of the common environmental allergens and some of the procedures that may be used to reduce exposure to them.

Dust Mites

Dust mites are microscopic members of the spider family. They live in places that are thick and hold moisture, such as mattresses, pillows, stuffed animals, and carpeting. A dusty shelf is not the problem. The allergen from the dust mites actually comes from their stool; their fecal pellets are about the same size as a pollen grain. The stools from the dust mites do not fly around easily, so they are usually a problem when the nose and mouth are near certain items. Exposure is increased when your child cuddles a stuffed animal, puts his head onto a pillow, or rolls around on carpeting or upholstered furniture. Dust mites would not float around an undisturbed room. Using special allergy-proof covers for bedding, mattresses, and pillows can reduce exposure to mites relatively easily. By enclosing bedding in these covers, the dust mite protein cannot be released and also the dust mite loses one source of food—the skin scales of humans. Some people recommend the removal of carpeting, although the above description may argue otherwise if your child is not spending a lot of time on the carpet. Reducing humidity, on which they need to live, and using hot water washes of bed linens, which kills them, are additional helpful measures to reduce exposure.

Molds

Mold, or fungus, can live indoors or outdoors. Molds may be a seasonal outdoor allergen or they may be an indoor allergen. In regard to the indoor exposure to molds, the places to consider are moist areas. Basement walls may develop a black or green discoloration that would indicate mold. A musty odor indicates mold growth. In bathrooms or kitchens, you may see some discoloration of the grout if there is mold contamination. Sometimes there are black, orange, or green circles of discoloration, or the shower curtains are discolored. If you have carpeting in your basement, you are essentially a mold farmer because you are giving mold a damp spot to grow. To reduce mold growth, reduce moisture. Use a dehumidifier, repair water leaks, and use special cleaners or weak chlorine solutions to combat mold.

Furry Pets

Cats, dogs, rabbits, gerbils, hamsters, mice, and other furry pets are a common indoor allergen. While some studies show that growing up with furry pets may reduce allergy risk, it is also true that children with pet allergies may suffer if their exposure continues. Unlike with dust mites, the protein that emanates from cats or dogs can become airborne quite easily and travel on small particles in the air that can be breathed deep into the lung, possibly causing sudden asthma for some sensitive individuals. Studies show that protein from cats, for example, is quite tenacious and can remain in homes even for weeks and months after a cat has been removed; so the removal of cat protein and possibly protein from other furred pets would require significant amounts of cleaning and washing, including wiping walls, shampooing carpets, and cleaning upholstered furniture. Studies typically do not show much success in trying to reduce exposure to cat protein if the cat is not removed from the home. The protein that emanates from furred pets typically comes from the saliva and oily secretions from the skin of these animals. Therefore, whether the animal sheds or has long hair or short hair typically does not affect its allergic potential.

Cockroach

Various emanations from cockroach are potentially allergenic. Studies show that if cockroaches are in the home, and the child who is allergic to cockroaches has asthma, there is an increased risk for more asthma-related illness. The removal of cockroaches from an apartment building could be very difficult because roaches travel easily from one apartment to the next, finding safe refuge. Remediation in this type of setting would require widespread extermination. It is usually easier to exterminate cockroaches from single-family homes. Keep food sources out of reach of these pests. This means keeping garbage closed, not having dirty dishes in the sink overnight, and sealing openings around pipes and other entry areas.

Pollens

Pollens derive from trees, grasses, and weeds. Airborne or windborne pollens that fly through the air in large concentrations are associated with allergies. This is different from flowers from florist shops which are brightly colored and transfer their pollen through insects. The pollens on these types of decorative plants, such as roses, are heavy, sticky, and tend not to become airborne; so unless you are a florist, it is not so likely that you would be allergic to them. However, the abundant pollen that emerges seasonally from trees, grass, and weeds poses significant issues for people with seasonal allergies. The specific season of pollination varies from location to location, so you should check with your allergist or pediatrician regarding your child's specific pollen allergies and the time of year that your child may have problems. If your child has a seasonal pollen allergy, medications can be started just prior to the pollen season, even before the problem starts. To reduce exposure to the pollens, keep windows closed and reduce outdoor activities when the pollen counts are high, which usually occurs on breezy, dry days. Children should wash their hands after playing outdoors to avoid touching their eyes when their hands are covered with pollen.

Insect Sting Allergy

Stinging insects, such as bees, yellow jackets, fire ants, and wasps, inject venom when they sting. Chemicals in the venom can cause pain and swelling, but it is also possible to be allergic to venom protein. Physicians usually do not screen a child in advance to determine whether they are venom-allergic because, like a food allergy, you may find a positive test that does not indicate a true allergic reaction. However, there are tests available for insect sting venoms, and if your child has experienced any type of significant allergic reaction from an insect sting, you should discuss this in detail with your allergist. Depending on the type of reaction that occurred, it may be useful to have a test conducted to confirm an allergy. Depending on the particular circumstances of the reaction and the test results, your allergist may recommend insect venom immunotherapy, or allergy shots. If your child has had a significant allergic reaction to an insect sting, the risk of another significant reaction is about 50 percent; but if your child is placed on allergy immunotherapy treatments for insect sting allergy, this risk would be reduced to less than 2 percent. Whether your child qualifies for this treatment should be discussed with your doctor.

Latex Allergy

Latex is a component of rubber products and is derived from the "rubber tree." Latex can be part of soft rubber products, such as rubber gloves, or hard rubber products, such as a rubber tire. When the latex is in a soft form, such as a rubber glove, it is easier for the latex to come off and trigger allergic reactions. Because latex is a product of nature, it is not a surprise that it shares many allergenic proteins with other items from nature. In particular, latex proteins are similar to the proteins of kiwi, avocado, and chestnut. A subset of people with latex allergy may react to these fruits, and a subset of people with these food allergies may have a problem with latex. In past years, it has primarily been individuals who have had repetitive surgeries or people who work in the health care field, that have been at the highest risk for developing a latex allergy. Because of the reduced use of these products, latex allergy has declined. Latex is sometimes used in sticky substances such as adhesive patches. If you suspect your child has a latex allergy, talk to your physician. Usually there is less concern about casual contact with latex in balls or balloons, than exposure to latex during major surgery. However, it is possible to have latex-free surgical operations. If your child experienced allergic symptoms with contact with rubber balloons or other rubber products, you should discuss this with your doctor because avoiding latex may be necessary.

Selected References

The material in this book is based on primary sources in the medical literature and clinical experience. The following list of medical references includes several key research and medical articles that review specific topics in food allergy. This list comprises only a portion of research articles on which discussions in this book are based. Although these articles are written for physicians, they may provide additional information on particular topics of interest for parents.

Altschul AS, Scherrer DL, Muñoz-Furlong A, Sicherer SH. Manufacturing and labeling issues for commercial products: Relevance to food allergy. *Journal of Allergy and Clinical Immunology.* 2001;108:468.

American Academy of Pediatrics. Committee on Nutrition. Hypoallergenic infant formulas. *Pediatrics.* 2000;106(2 pt 1):346–349.

Bernstein IL, Storms WW. Practice parameters for allergy diagnostic testing. Joint Task Force on Practice Parameters for the Diagnosis and Treatment of Asthma. American Academy of Allergy, Asthma and Immunology and the American College of Allergy, Asthma and Immunology. *Annals of Allergy, Asthma & Immunology.* 1995;75(6 pt 2): 543–625.

Beyer K, Morrow E, Li XM, Bardina L, Bannon GA, Burks AW, et al. Effects of cooking methods on peanut allergenicity. *Journal of Allergy and Clinical Immunology.* 2001; 107(6):1077–1081.

Bock SA, Muñoz-Furlong A, Sampson HA. Fatalities due to anaphylactic reactions to foods. *Journal of Allergy and Clinical Immunology.* 2001;107(1):191–193.

Burks AW, Bannon GA, Sicherer SH, Sampson HA. Peanut-induced anaphylaxis. *International Archives of Allergy and Immunology.* 1999;119:165–172.

Busse PJ, Noone SA, Nowak-Wegrzyn AH, Sampson HA, Sicherer SH. Recurrent peanut allergy. *New England Journal Medicine.* 2002;347:1535–1356.

Chapman JA, Bernstein IL, Lee RE, et al. Food allergy: A practice parameter. *Annals of Allergy, Asthma & Immunology.* 2006;96:S1–S68.

Cohen BL, Noone S, Muñoz-Furlong A, Sicherer SH. Development of a questionnaire to measure quality of life in families with a food-allergic child. *Journal of Allergy and Clinical Immunology.* 2004;114(5):1159–1163.

Derby CJ, Gowland MH, Hourihane JO. Sesame allergy in Britain: A questionnaire survey of members of the Anaphylaxis Campaign. *Pediatric Allergy and Immunology.* 2005;16(2):171–175.

Eigenmann PA, Sicherer SH, Borkowski TA, Cohen BA, Sampson HA. Prevalence of IgE-mediated food allergy among children with atopic dermatitis. *Pediatrics.* 1998; 101:E8.

Fleischer DM, Conover-Walker MK, Christie L, Burks AW, Wood RA. The natural progression of peanut allergy: Resolution and the possibility of recurrence. *Journal of Allergy and Clinical Immunology.* 2003;112(1):183–189.

Furlong TJ, DeSimone J, Sicherer SH. Peanut and tree nut allergic reactions in restaurants and other food establishments. *Journal of Allergy and Clinical Immunology.* 2001;108:867–870.

Hefle SL, Nordlee JA, Taylor SL. Allergenic foods. *Critical Reviews in Food Science and Nutrition.* 1996;36(suppl):S69–S89.

Hsieh KY, Tsai CC, Wu CH, Lin RH. Epicutaneous exposure to protein antigen and food allergy. *Clinical and Experimental Allergy.* 2003;33(8):1067–1075.

Joshi P, Mofidi S, Sicherer SH. Interpretation of commercial food ingredient labels by parents of food allergic children. *Journal of Allergy and Clinical Immunology.* 2002;109:1019–1021.

Lack G, Fox D, Northstone K, Golding J. Factors associated with the development of peanut allergy in childhood. *New England Journal of Medicine.* 2003;348(11):977–985.

Leung DYM, Sampson HA, Yunginger JW, Burks W, Schneider LC, Shanahan W. Effect of anti-IgE therapy (TNX-901) in patients with severe peanut allergy. *New England Journal of Medicine.* 2003;348:986–993.

Ma S, Sicherer SH, Nowak-Wegrzyn A. A survey on the management of pollen-food allergy syndrome (OAS) in allergy practices. *Journal of Allergy and Clinical Immunology.* 2003;112:784–788.

Mofidi SM. Nutritional management of pediatric food hypersensitivity. *Pediatrics.* 2003;111:1645–1653.

Muraro A, Dreborg S, Halken S, Host A, Niggemann B, Aalberse R, et al. Dietary prevention of allergic diseases in infants and small children. Part 3: Critical review of published peer-reviewed observational and interventional studies and final recommendations. *Pediatric Allergy and Immunology.* 2004;15(4):291–307.

Nowak-Wegrzyn A, Conover-Walker MK, Wood RA. Food-allergic reactions in schools and preschools. *Archives of Pediatrics & Adolescent Medicine.* 2001;155(7):790–795.

Nowak-Wegrzyn A, Sampson HA. Food allergy therapy. *Immunology and Allergy Clinics of North America.* 2004;24(4):705–725.

Nowak-Wegrzyn A, Sampson HA, Wood RA, Sicherer SH. Food protein-induced enterocolitis syndrome caused by solid food proteins. *Pediatrics.* 2003;111:829–835.

Perry TT, Conover-Walker MK, Pomes A, Chapman MD, Wood RA. Distribution of peanut allergen in the environment. *Journal of Allergy and Clinical Immunology.* 2004;113(5):973–976.

Perry TT, Matsui EC, Kay Conover-Walker M, Wood RA. The relationship of allergen-specific IgE levels and oral food challenge outcome. *Journal of Allergy and Clinical Immunology.* 2004;114(1):144–149.

Rothenberg ME, Mishra A, Collins MH, Putnam PE. Pathogenesis and clinical features of eosinophilic esophagitis. *Journal of Allergy and Clinical Immunology.* 2001; 108(6):891–894.

Sampson HA. Update on food allergy. *Journal of Allergy and Clinical Immunology.* 2004; 113(5):805–819.

Sampson HA. Utility of food-specific IgE concentrations in predicting symptomatic food allergy. *Journal of Allergy and Clinical Immunology.* 2001;107(5):891–896.

Sampson HA, Mendelson LM, Rosen JP. Fatal and near-fatal anaphylactic reactions to food in children and adolescents. *New England Journal of Medicine.* 1992;327:380–384.

Sampson HA, Muñoz-Furlong A, Bock SA, et al. Symposium on the definition and management of anaphylaxis: summary report. *Journal of Allergy and Clinical Immunology.* 2005;115(3):584–591.

Sampson HA, Sicherer SH. Eczema and food hypersensitivity. *Immunology and Allergy Clinics of North America.* 1999;19:495–517.

Sampson HA, Sicherer SH, Birnbaum A. AGA technical review on the evaluation of food allergy in gastrointestinal disorders. *Gastroenterology.* 2001;120:1026–1040.

Shreffler WG, Beyer K, Chu TH, Burks AW, Sampson HA. Microarray immunoassay: association of clinical history, in vitro IgE function, and heterogeneity of allergenic peanut epitopes. *Journal of Allergy and Clinical Immunology.* 2004;113(4):776–782.

Sicherer SH. Beyond oral food challenges: improved modalities to diagnose food hypersensitivity disorders. *Current Opinion in Allergy and Clinical Immunology.* 2003; 3:185–188.

Sicherer SH. Clinical aspects of gastrointestinal food allergy in childhood. *Pediatrics.* 2003;111:1609–1616.

Sicherer SH. Clinical implications of cross-reacting food proteins. *Journal of Allergy and Clinical Immunology.* 2001;108:881–890.

Sicherer SH. Diagnosis and management of childhood food allergy. *Current Problems in Pediatrics.* 2001;31:35–57.

Sicherer SH. Food allergy. *Lancet.* 2002;360:701–710.

Sicherer SH. Food challenges: when and how to perform oral food challenges. *Pediatric Allergy and Immunology.* 1999;10:226–234.

Sicherer SH. Food protein-induced enterocolitis syndrome: case presentations and management lessons. *Journal of Allergy and Clinical Immunology.* Jan 2005;115(1):149–156.

Sicherer SH. Food protein-induced enterocolitis syndrome: clinical perspectives. *Journal of Pediatric Gastroenterology and Nutrition.* 2000;30:S45–S49.

Sicherer SH. The genetics of food allergy. *Immunology and Allergy Clinics of North America.* 2002;22:211–222.

Sicherer SH. The impact of maternal diet during breast feeding on the prevention of food allergy. *Current Opinion in Allergy and Clinical Immunology.* 2002;2:207–210.

Sicherer SH. Is food allergy causing your patient's asthma symptoms? *Journal of Respiratory Diseases.* 2000;21:127–136.

Sicherer SH. Manifestations of food allergy: diagnosis and treatment. *American Family Physician.* 1998;59:415–424.

Sicherer SH. New insights on the natural history of peanut allergy [editorial]. *Annals of Allergy, Asthma & Immunology.* 2000;85:435–437.

Sicherer SH. Peanut allergy: a clinical update. *Annals of Allergy, Asthma & Immunology.* 2002;88:350–361.

Sicherer SH. Self-injectable epinephrine: one size does not fit all [editorial]. *Annals of Allergy, Asthma & Immunology.* 2001;86:597–598.

Sicherer SH. Systemic aspects of food allergy. *Journal of Allergy and Clinical Immunology.* 2000;106:S251–S257.

Sicherer SH, Burks AW, Sampson HA. Clinical features of acute allergic reactions to peanut and tree nuts in children. *Pediatrics.* 1998;102:E6.

Sicherer SH, Burks AW, Sampson HA. Peanut and soy allergy: a diagnostic and therapeutic dilemma. *Allergy.* 2000;55:515–521.

Sicherer SH, Eigenmann PA, Sampson HA. Clinical features of food protein-induced enterocolitis syndrome. *Journal of Pediatrics.* 1998;133:214–219.

Sicherer SH, Forman JA, Noone SA. Use assessment of self-administered epinephrine among food allergic children and pediatricians. *Pediatrics.* 2000;105:359–362.

Sicherer SH, Furlong TJ, DeSimone J, Sampson HA. Peanut allergic reactions in schools. *Journal of Pediatrics.* 2001;138:56–55.

Sicherer SH, Furlong TJ, DeSimone J, Sampson HA. Self-reported peanut allergic reactions on commercial airlines. *Journal of Allergy and Clinical Immunology.* 1999; 104:186–189.

Sicherer SH, Furlong T, Maes HH, Desnick RJ, Sampson HA, Gelb BD. Genetics of peanut allergy: a twin study. *Journal of Allergy and Clinical Immunology.* 2000;106:53–56.

Sicherer SH, Furlong TJ, Muñoz-Furlong A, Burks AW, Sampson HA. A Voluntary registry for peanut and tree nut allergy: characteristics of the first 5,149 registrants. *Journal of Allergy and Clinical Immunology.* 2001;108:138–142.

Sicherer SH, Morrow EH, Sampson HA. Dose-response in double-blind, placebo-controlled food challenges in children with atopic dermatitis. *Journal of Allergy and Clinical Immunology.* 2000;105:582–586.

Sicherer SH, Muñoz-Furlong A, Burks AW, Sampson HA. Prevalence of peanut and tree nut allergy in the U.S. determined by a random digit dial telephone survey. *Journal of Allergy and Clinical Immunology.* 1999;103:559–562.

Sicherer SH, Muñoz-Furlong A, Murphy R, Wood RA, Sampson HA. Symposium: pediatric food allergy. *Pediatrics.* 2003;111:1591–1594.

Sicherer SH, Muñoz-Furlong A, Sampson HA. Prevalence of peanut and tree nut allergy in the U.S. determined by a random digit dial telephone survey: a five-year follow-up Study. *Journal of Allergy and Clinical Immunology.* 2003;112:1203–1207.

Sicherer SH, Muñoz-Furlong A, Sampson HA. Prevalence of seafood allergy in the United States determined by a random telephone survey. *Journal of Allergy and Clinical Immunology.* 2004;114:159–165.

Sicherer SH, Noone SA, Barnes-Koerner C, Christie L, Burks AW, Sampson HA. Hypoallergenicity and efficacy of an amino acid–based formula in children with cow's milk and multiple food hypersensitivities. *Journal of Pediatrics.* 2001;138:688–693.

Sicherer SH, Noone SA, Muñoz-Furlong A. The impact of childhood food allergy on quality of life. *Annals of Allergy, Asthma & Immunology.* 2001;87:461–464.

Sicherer SH, Sampson HA. Auriculotemporal syndrome: a masquerader of food allergy. *Journal of Allergy and Clinical Immunology.* 1996;97:851–852.

Sicherer SH, Sampson HA. Cow's milk protein-specific IgE concentrations in two age groups of milk-allergic children and in children achieving clinical tolerance. *Clinical and Experimental Allergy.* 1999;29:507–512.

Sicherer SH, Sampson, HA. Food allergy. *Journal of Allergy and Clinical Immunology.* 2006;117:5470–5475.

Sicherer SH, Sampson HA. Food hypersensitivity and atopic dermatitis: pathophysiology, epidemiology, diagnosis, and management. *Journal of Allergy and Clinical Immunology.* 1999;104:114–122.

Sicherer SH, Sampson HA. The role of food allergy in childhood asthma. *Immunology and Allergy Clinics of North America.* 1998;18:49–60.

Sicherer SH, Sampson HA. Peanut and tree nut allergy. *Current Opinion in Pediatrics.* 2000;12:567–573.

Sicherer SH, Simons FER. Quandaries in prescribing an emergency action plan and self-injectable epinephrine for first aid management of anaphylaxis in the community. *Journal of Allergy and Clinical Immunology.* 2005;115:575–583.

Sicherer SH, Teuber SS. Academy practice paper: current approach to the diagnosis and management of adverse reactions to foods. *Journal of Allergy and Clinical Immunology.* 2004;114(5):1146–1150.

Simons E, Weiss C, Furlong T, Sicherer SH. Impact of ingredient labeling practices on food-allergic consumers. *Annals of Allergy, Asthma & Immunology.* 2005;95:426–428.

Simonte SJ, Ma S, Mofidi S, Sicherer SH. Relevance of casual contact to peanut butter in peanut-allergic children. *Journal of Allergy and Clinical Immunology.* 2003;112:180–183.

Vadas P, Wai Y, Burks W, Perelman B. Detection of peanut allergens in breast milk of lactating women. *Journal of the American Medical Association.* 2001;285(13):1746–1748.

Wang J, Sicherer SH. Anaphylaxis following ingestion of candy fruit chews. *Annals of Allergy, Asthma & Immunology.* May 2005;94(5):530–533.

Wood RA. The natural history of food allergy. *Pediatrics.* 2003;111(6 pt 3):1631–1637.

Zeiger RS, Heller S. The development and prediction of atopy in high-risk children: follow-up at age 7 years in a prospective randomized study of combined maternal and infant food allergen avoidance. *Journal of Allergy and Clinical Immunology.* 1995;95(6): 1179–1790.

Index

ABOUT THE AUTHOR

Scott H. Sicherer, M.D., is associate professor of Pediatrics at the Mount Sinai School of Medicine and a researcher in the Jaffe Food Allergy Institute at Mount Sinai. Dr. Sicherer received his medical degree with honors from the Johns Hopkins University School of Medicine, and his pediatric training, including a chief residency, at Mount Sinai in New York City. He completed a Fellowship in Allergy and Immunology at Johns Hopkins and then returned as faculty to Mt. Sinai. He is board certified in pediatrics and in allergy and immunology and specializes in food allergies.

His research interests, funded by the National Institutes of Health, U.S. Department of Agriculture, Food Allergy Initiative, and the Food Allergy & Anaphylaxis Network, include allergic diseases caused by specific foods such as peanuts, tree nuts, eggs, seafood, and milk; the natural history of food allergy; atopic dermatitis; gastrointestinal manifestations of food allergies; epidemiology of food allergy; psychosocial issues associated with food allergies; modalities to educate physicians and parents about food allergy; and the genetics of food allergy.

Dr. Sicherer has published more than 100 articles in scientific journals, including the *Journal of Allergy and Clinical Immunology, Pediatrics, New England Journal of Medicine,* the *Journal of the American Medical Association, Lancet, Clinical and Experimental Allergy, Journal of Pediatrics,* and many others. He has authored numerous book chapters in major pediatric and allergy textbooks. He is a medical advisor to the Food Allergy & Anaphylaxis Network, the Food Allergy Initiative, and others. He is past-chair of the Adverse Reactions to Foods Committee of the Academy of Allergy, Asthma and Immunology. He is associate editor of the *Journal of Allergy and Clinical Immunology.* Dr. Sicherer has authored a children's book on food allergy, *Maya and Andrew Learn about Food Allergies,* and co-authored a book about peanut allergy, *The Complete Peanut Allergy Handbook.*

Consistently recognized as a top doctor by Castle-Connolly/*New York Magazine,* he lectures extensively on food allergy topics to various professional and lay organizations. He has had numerous television and radio appearances to discuss food allergy.

Dr. Scott Sicherer, his wife, and their five children reside in New Jersey.